350
BEST SEX
TIPS EVER

SATISFACTION GUARANTEED

THIS IS A CARLTON BOOK

Text, illustrations and design copyright © 2003
Carlton Books Limited
This edition published by Carlton Books Limited 2003
20 Mortimer Street, London W1T 3JW

Reprinted in 2008

A CIP catalogue record for this book is available from
the British Library.
ISBN-13 978 1 84442 912 7

Printed in Singapore

Editorial Manager: **Judith More**
Art Director: **Penny Stock**
Executive Editor: **Lisa Dyer**
Copy Editors: **Jane Donovan and Toria Leitch**
Design: **DW Design**
Production Controller: **Lucy Woodhead**
Illustrator: **Nicola Slater**

Neither the author nor the publisher can accept responsibility for any
accident, injury or damage that results from using the ideas, information
or advice offered in this book.

350
BEST SEX
TIPS EVER

SATISFACTION GUARANTEED

LISA SUSSMAN

CARLTON
BOOKS

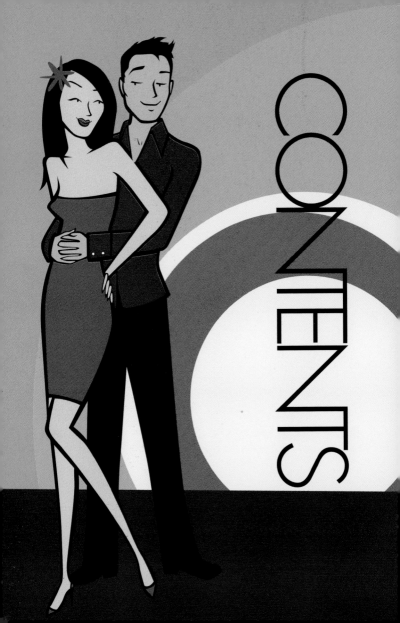

CONTENTS

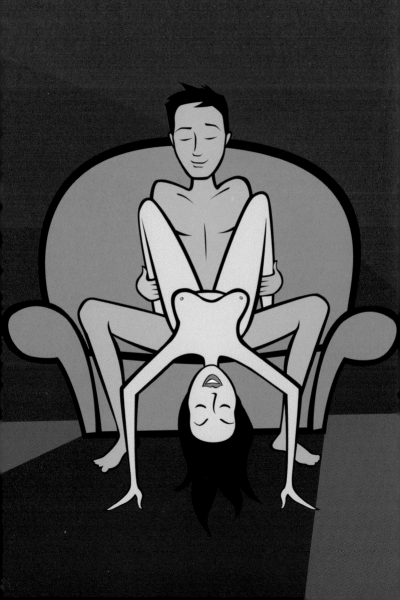

SEX POSITIONS

OVER 100 TRULY EXPLOSIVE TIPS

RATINGS

To give you some guidelines, some of the following positions have been road tested and rated as follows:

Getting it Right

 Easy peasy.

 Read the directions carefully.

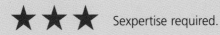 Sexpertise required.

Orgasmic Potential

 Sweet comfortable screw.

 A bit of a body rattler.

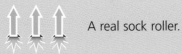 A real sock roller.

1

Erotic Sex

In other words, enjoying happy horizontal hula simply for pleasure's sake.

SEX POSITION TIPS

Don't just settle for missionary monotony! Whether you're stuck in a sexual rut or just eager for some between-the-sheets experimentation, here's the ultimate guide to positioning yourself (and your partner) for the best sex ever. Let the games begin!

TAKE UP YOUR POSITIONS …

For some **triple X-rated** twists on the old in and out.

MAN ON TOP (AKA 'MISSIONARY')
The Old Move: The classic man on top, woman beneath him, face-to-face position. He supports weight on his arms and you straddle his hips with your legs. It's great for easy thrusting (him) and creating close, intimate contact between you.

Make It Better: Do the knee–chest. Raise your legs so that your knees are pressed to your chest, then drape your legs over his shoulders. This will make your vagina longer, which will make his toes curl because he can penetrate you more deeply and give you more friction and pressure where you crave it most – on your vaginal lips and clitoris.

WOMAN ON TOP

The Old Move: This lets you stay in control and show your stuff. Simply sit on his penis and rotate those hips! Sitting is for sex in slow motion – the angles are all wrong for any sort of energetic thrusting. The man either sits in a chair or cross-legged on the floor, while you sit astride him, usually face to face, although it can work equally well if you face away from him. This position is good for caressing and intimacy.

Make It Better: Face his toes instead of his head. Then, as you lift yourself up and down, rotate your body in small circles. Tease him by using your vaginal lips to rub his erect penis – tantalize him by degrees until he's squirming.

★ ★

3

STANDING

The Old Move: Standing is best for quickie trysts, but if he's much taller than you it's difficult to manage as he has to hold you up or you have to stand on a stool so his penis can reach your vagina.

Make It Better: Turn around and lean over to give him a delicious view of your derrière. Lift one leg sideways so he can slip inside you without having to twist, then close your legs slightly so he doesn't pop out. His hands can slip around to your clitoris to add a little extra heat.

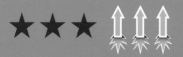

SIDE BY SIDE (AKA 'SPOONING')

The Old Move: Side by side is a lovely cuddly move that's perfect for canoodling. The classic is spooning (lying on your side facing away from him so that he enters you from behind with his arms wrapped around you).

Make It Better: Have your lover lie on his back. Then, facing away from him, lower your crotch onto his (your arms should be stretched out behind you to support your weight). He encircles your waist with his legs and grips your thighs. Then you both roll over together onto your sides. He can then thrust gently into you …

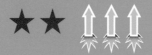

REAR ENTRY (AKA 'DOGGIE')

The Old Move: The classic doggie-style position is a pleasure howler that gives ultra-deep penetration. You kneel on all fours and he slips in from behind …

Make It Better: Your partner lies on his back with a pillow beneath his head so he can watch all the action. Facing his feet, you straddle him. Then, placing your hands on the floor first, you back onto his penis. He holds your thighs or buttocks tightly while you thrust up and down the entire length of him. This is doing it doggie your way – you have maximum control while your partner gets to savour every sensation without working up too much sweat. It's a fantastic position for a truly intense G-spot orgasm.

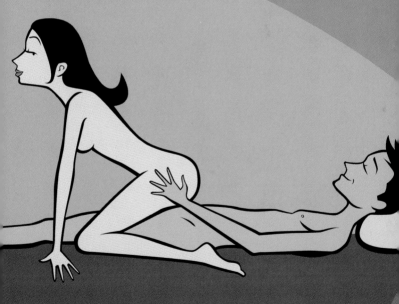

PUSH YOUR BUTTONS …

It still comes as a constant surprise to most guys, but intercourse isn't the best way for them to push you over the edge. Here's how to get him to trigger your orgasm switch.

HIT THE C NOTE

The clitoris is your hot button to bliss! Sex researcher Shere Hite found that over 75 per cent of women need to have this little bit of flesh stimulated in order to orgasm during sex.

- Doggie-style sex leaves his hands free to go walkies all over your breasts and clitoris (see tip 5).

- Twirling his penis around inside your vagina will slide it against your vaginal walls while his pubic bone grinds against your clitoris. You lie face up on the floor with a couple of pillows propping up your behind. Keep your knees half-bent, your legs splayed and your arms high above your head. Your partner enters you from a high angle, planting his hands on the floor beside your head. He moves around inside you in slow figure-of-eight motions.

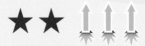

- Putting your feet on his buttocks when you're in missionary mode will graze his pubic bone against your clitoris. Double your pleasure by raising your legs – the higher you lift them, the deeper the penetration against the front wall of your vagina, which is where your G-spot is.
- Spreading a little water-based KY Jelly on his penis, climbing on top of him (but without putting him inside you) and then moving back and forth will put enticing pressure on your clitoris.
- Lying on your back with your legs shut adds stimulation to your clitoris, and allows more friction with the nerve-rich surface of your vagina (not to mention his penis).
- To hit your clitoris every time – MEOW! – try the coital alignment technique (also known as the CAT). Instead of entering you straight on in the missionary position, he rides high so that his pubic bone – the hard surface just above the shaft of his penis – applies pressure to the rounded bit above your vagina (the hood) where the clitoris hides. Settling into a gentle mutual rhythm in which he rocks his pubic bone back and forth over your clitoris, rather than focusing so much on thrusting in and out, you get stimulated in all the right places.

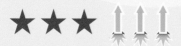

G IS FOR GLORIOUS-ASM!

(7)

Researcher Beverly Whipple discovered that
halfway up the front wall of your vagina is
a soft swelling that will make you scream with
joy whenever it's pressed. These positions hit
the G-spot's bull's-eye every time:

- Sitting on top of him, facing his feet.
- Get on top and lean backwards and forwards.
- You lie on your stomach while he gently lies on
  top of you so he can penetrate you deeply from
  behind. You'll get G-
  spot and clitoral sparks
  at the same time!
- Get underneath him and
  have him place his hands beneath
  your hips and lift your whole pelvic
  area into the air.

GO TO YOUR AFE ZONE

The anterior fornix erogenous is located on the front wall of the vagina, a third of the way down from the cervix. Studies have found that 95 per cent of women had not only the most orgasms, but also the most intense ones of their lives when this area was caressed. Try these tips:

- Rear entry is the best move for hitting your Aaah ... zone (see tip 5).
- Slipping a pillow underneath your hips when you're on the bottom tilts your pelvis forward and has the same effect.
- Lie on your back at the end of the bed and have him stand between your legs.
- Get into the missionary position (see tip 1) and hook your ankles around his shoulders or neck.
- When your AFE area is hit, this can result in waves of muscular contractions that seem hellbent on pushing your lover right out of you. When this happens, get him to push back. The more he pushes into you forcefully, the more intense your pleasure will be.

PENIS TICKLERS

These moves will make sure you give his favourite organ a total va-va-voom buzz during sex.

Whenever you're **on top of him**, facing his feet, consider this little trick: just as he's about to have his orgasm, grasp his toes and pull gently. It seems that the nerves in his toes are connected to the ones in his genitals so this extra stimulation increases the intensity of his ejaculation.

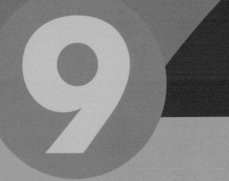

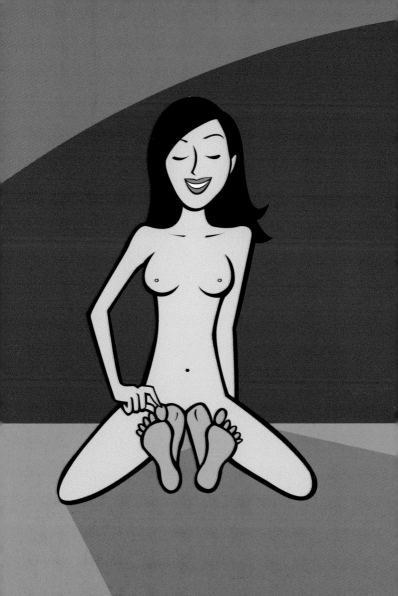

While on top (see tip 2), keep his penile skin **stretched tight** by holding it down at the base with your fingers. Imagine the heightened sensitivity you would experience if he stretched the skin around your exposed clitoris while thrusting against it with his pelvis and you'll understand why this manoeuvre can send him skyward!

When he's lying on top of you during sex, get him to **spread his legs** to take the pressure away from his testicles. If too compressed, they may become understimulated.

Lie flat on top of him with your legs in between his and squeeze your thighs tightly together. This way, you get to control how deeply he penetrates you while tantalizing the packed-with-nerve-endings head of his penis.

Double his pleasure by turning on his **G-spot**. When you're on top (see tip 2) or underneath (see tip 1), reach behind and press on the area between his backside and balls with your forefinger.

His penis is never happier than when it's **sliding inside** you as deeply as he possibly can. To give him the ground zero penetration, get into the missionary position (see tip 1) and lift your legs up and apart. The higher you can go, the further he'll be able to thrust – especially if you push into him with each stroke. (It helps if you wrap your legs around his shoulders.)

Sit up straight on top of him – you can face either way to do this. Now grind your pelvis around and around, back and forth. At the same time, squeeze your vaginal muscles tight until you vibrate him into sex heaven.

GET SYNCHRONIZED!

For a move even yummier than a five-star French meal, master the *soixante-neuf*.

16

Ask him to **hum** while he's giving you oral pleasure with his tongue on your pleasure knob.

17

Do the **60-minute** lick.
Ask for one slow, long, wet lick around your clitoris and return the favour on his love stick.

18

To prevent yourself from **gagging** while pleasuring him, hold the base of his penis as you suck. You'll control how deeply his penis thrusts into your mouth.

Up his pleasure! Play with his nipples or massage his buttocks.

19

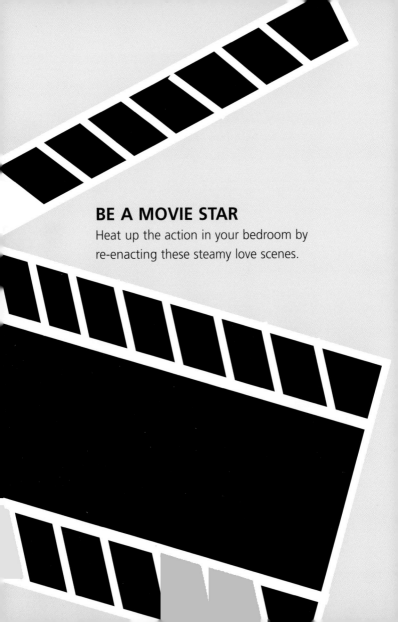

BE A MOVIE STAR

Heat up the action in your bedroom by re-enacting these steamy love scenes.

20

NINE AND A HALF WEEKS

Fill your fridge with lots of sticky, squishy and yummy foods like strawberries, grapes, ice cream, chocolate mousse and orange juice. Take it in turns to blindfold each other and feed and drip the food over every orifice, alternating with tips 2, 5 AND 16–19).

21

OUT OF SIGHT

Substitute the car boot (trunk) for any cramped, dark space (a closet will do). Slip into a short, business-like dress, then jam your bodies together on the floor in a spoon position (see tip 4). He starts off by languidly stroking your thigh before roaming over the rest of your body.

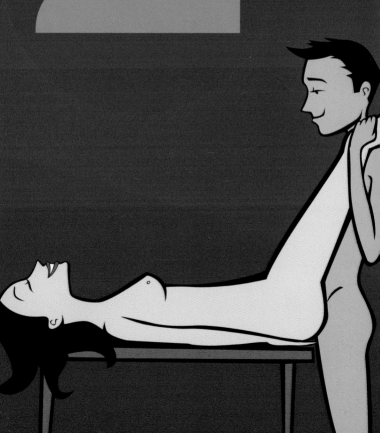

THE POSTMAN ALWAYS RINGS TWICE

Sweep away everything from the kitchen table. Lie down on your back at the edge, extend your legs straight up, keeping them close together, and put your hands underneath your buttocks to elevate your pelvis. Standing up and gripping your legs for leverage and stability, your partner then enters you.

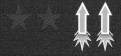

STRETCH IT OUT!

The looser and more supple your muscles, the more moves you can make. These stretches will help limber you into a sex gymnast!

POWER SQUATS

For overall improved **hip strength** and flexibility, stand with your feet slightly more than shoulder width apart and your arms straight out in front of you for balance. Bring your hips and backside back, bend your knees forward (no farther than your toes) and then straighten your legs. Do three sets of 15 repetitions a week.

BODY DIPS

Strengthen your triceps so that you can hold yourself up for longer periods when you're on top (see tip 2). Sit on a sturdy chair with its back securely against a wall. Hold the front of the seat on each side of your legs with the heels of your hands. Slide gently off the chair and pose, knees bent, with your elbows pointing towards the wall and your arms supporting your body. Lower your body, bending your elbows to a 90-degree angle and then push up. Do three sets of 15 repetitions a week.

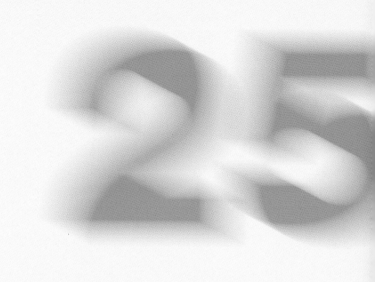

HIP STRETCH

This exercise improves your **range of motion** when you're underneath (see tip 1). Lie on your back with your knees bent and your feet on the floor. Place your left foot comfortably across the middle of your right thigh, with your left thigh resting open. (For a better stretch, position your left foot closer to your hip.) Now pull your right thigh towards your chest for 20–30 seconds. Alternate sides for a total of three repetitions per side each week.

INNER THIGH AND HAMSTRING STRETCH

Limber yourself up for more athletic sexual positions. Sit **on the floor** with your legs pointing outwards in a 'V' position. For a wider stretch, place your hands behind you to support yourself and push your backside forwards, then lift it off the floor with small pelvic thrusts. Return to the start position, then turn your upper body towards one foot. Keeping your back as flat as possible, reach for that foot with your hands. Alternate sides for a total of three repetitions per side every week.

26

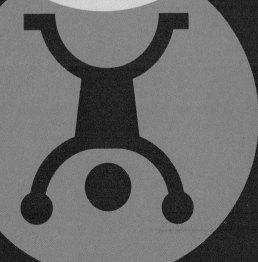

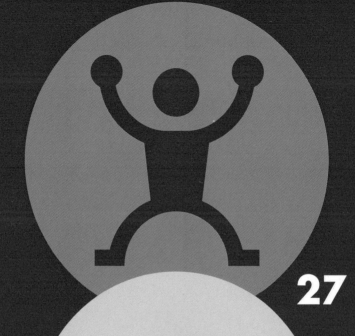

27

PC PUMPER

Strengthening your pubococcygeus (PC) muscles **enhances sexual pleasure**. Do this exercise regularly and you'll be able to milk his member to ecstasy while at the same time boosting your own orgasmic potential. Squeeze the muscles that control your urine flow for five seconds and then release. Do this for a minimum of 30 repetitions each day.

2

Sensual Sex

This is lovemaking that encompasses everything around you, so you slowly and steadily stimulate each other to intense peaks of sexual pleasure.

BEDROOM SEXESSORIES

Set the stage for your love ride …

28

Before making love, place **mirrors** all around your room so you can see your reflections from all angles. Stand up (see tip 3) so you can press your body up against your reflection and get the erotic boost of seemingly making love to yourself.

29

Slip onto a luxurious **fur throw** or thick, soft rug to make love. The material feels very sensual to naked bodies.

All **fabrics** in the bedroom should be invitingly tactile – soft cotton, smooth silk, rich velvet, cool satin and knobbly bedspreads (for delicious friction).

Lightly **scent the room** or the sheets with a musky or flowery perfume. Everything else will smell fresh and clean. Eventually he'll begin to associate this scent with your lovemaking and you'll get him in the mood with just one whiff.

USE ALL YOUR SENSES

When you make love, indulge in a sensual feast.

Create the **sounds of seduction**. Have him get on top (see tip 1). Relax your vaginal muscles as he moves up and tighten them on the downswing. With practice, you'll make a loud, sexy, squishy sound. After orgasm, ask him to stretch out so he's lying flat on top of your body. The sound of his heartbeat will reverberate through your body.

Give the look of love. Sitting straight up on top of him gives you a sizzling full-eye view of each other.

Give off sexy scents. Slip into the missionary position (see tip 1) and lift your arms over your head to open your armpits (a sexy source of pheromones). One whiff will plunge you both into accelerated lust.

Indulge in a **tasty turn-on**. Lie on top of him so that your face is by his feet and your feet are by his head. Called a '20', this position lets you nibble each other's toes at the same time.

Discover the **power of touch**. Try making love in the dark. You have to feel your way, and not knowing where you'll be touched next can heighten the sexual tension. There's also something about being unable to see that makes your other senses respond more intensely to every sensation.

SLOW-HIM-DOWN SEX

Strike a pose and increase his staying power.

Change your position a few times during lovemaking. The momentary lapse can halt his momentum, which should curb early ejaculation.

Try the **Stop/Start Technique**. It doesn't matter what position you're in, but you should do most of the moving. With him lying as still as possible, gently move up and down until he nears his big moment. Stop if he's about to take an express trip to bliss until he's got himself in hand. But remember, thinking about something boring to delay ejaculation rarely works. Besides, it makes your love play slightly schizophrenic – you're turned on while he's obsessing about whether he can afford a new car! So, while all this stopping and starting is going on, he should be selfishly, happily and contentedly concentrating completely on his arousal. Once he can last as long as he wants to, he can start moving his hips as well.

Climbing on top and facing him (see tip 2) gives you total control over his – and your – sensations, especially if you ride your partner while kneeling or sitting. By keeping penetration shallow, you'll be able to set the pace as slow as you want without him jumping his orgasmic gun.

So long as he's at least **as tall as you**, you can have sex in a kneeling position, even if he isn't fully erect. He sits on the raised heels of his feet and you squat over him, face to face, with your thighs spread out. Now guide his penis inside you. Once he's in, you can take some of the weight off his back by leaning back on one arm while holding onto him with the other.

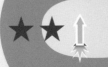

SLOW COMFORTABLE SCREWS

Well, you want this exquisite agony to go on for at least a few more hours, don't you?

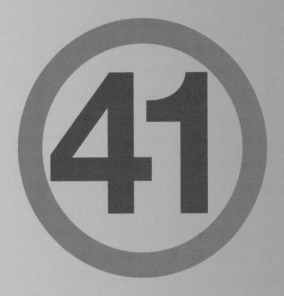

To **slow things down** a bit, get on top (see tip 2) or underneath (see tip 1). Completely relax your vaginal muscles and place your legs flat alongside his. This makes for shallower thrusts, but keep your hips rocking so your bodies know you're still interested.

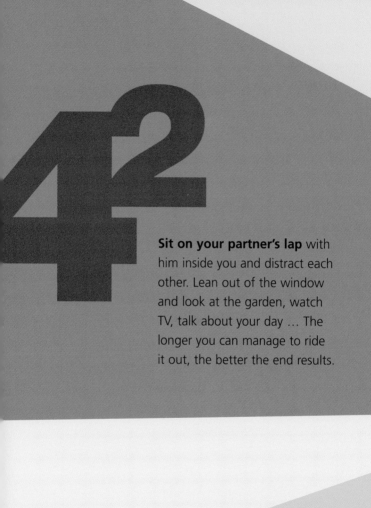

42

Sit on your partner's lap with him inside you and distract each other. Lean out of the window and look at the garden, watch TV, talk about your day ... The longer you can manage to ride it out, the better the end results.

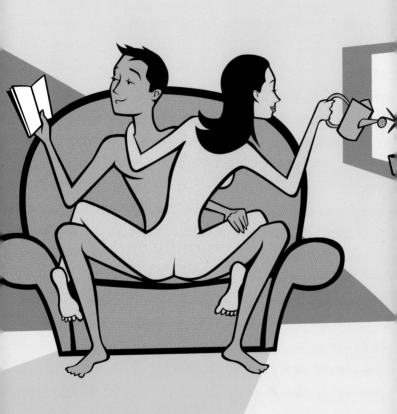

Moving in **slow motion** makes you acutely aware of every part of the movement, from the muscles and body parts you're using to your weight shifts and your breathing – all of which you miss when you move too fast. Slip into a relaxing, sensual move such as the sidestroke, with both of you lying on your sides and him curled up behind you. Tell him to insert his penis slowly while you both focus on the feeling of your skin making contact, on your breathing and on the pleasurable pressure of his penis as it advances, little by little. Take a full minute to perform what you would usually do in just one or two seconds. You'll need to towel off after this one!

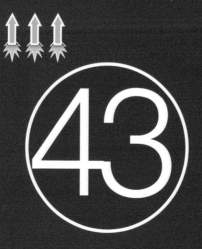

43

Get into **woman-on-top** mode (see tip 2), straddling his hips. Lower yourself onto his penis, but go no farther than the glans (the very tip of it). Then lift yourself back up in retreat and repeat nine times. On the tenth repetition, lower yourself all the way down onto his penis, letting him thrust fully into your vaginal canal. Pull yourself back up and begin your next set of attack and retreat, but this time allow eight shallow thrusts and two deep ones, followed by seven shallow and three deep thrusts, and so on. By the time you're taking ten deep thrusts from him, you'll have lost count. (If you don't have strong, steely thigh muscles, try leaning forward over your partner and use your abdominal muscles to lift your pelvis up and down until you collapse in delight.)

MOOD BUSTERS

Libido lift-offs, whatever your state of mind.

WHEN YOU'RE NEW LOVERS 45

For **first-time sex** – or first-time-together sex –
any position where he's on top (see tip 1) will
be the most comfortable and require the least
amount of effort from you (you have enough
to think about). Ease things along by placing
a pillow under your hips. Another tip you might
try is to push your pelvis down as he enters you
to help relax things down there.

WHEN YOU HAVE YOUR PERIOD

Assume **the spoon** (see tip 4). Then lift your
top leg while he shifts his lower body into a half-
kneeling position and enters you from behind.
This half-doggie, half-spooning hybrid combines
the cosy intimacy of lying side by side with G-spot-
rubbing rear entry without ever making an issue
of your period bloat.

46

47

WHEN YOU HAVE A HANGOVER

Getting the blood to rush straight to your head helps ease all that pounding, as will having a brain-melting orgasm. Studies show that an orgasm is the **best cure for a headache**. Start with your partner lying on his back. Facing his feet, straddle his hips on your knees and lower yourself onto his penis. Slowly extend your legs back towards his shoulders and relax your torso onto the bed or ground between his feet. Both sets of legs should now form an 'X' shape. Use your PC muscles (see tip 27) and move your buttocks up and down or back and forth to maintain his erection.

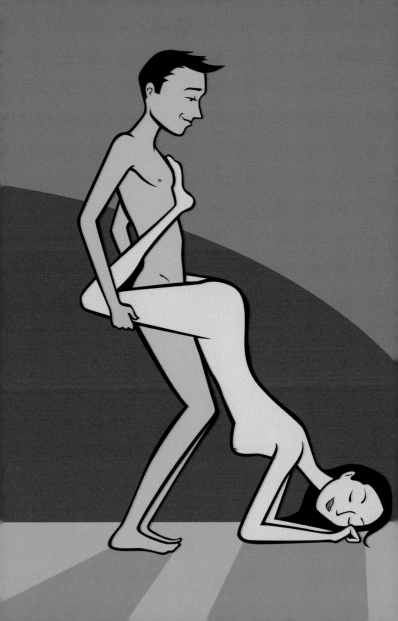

48

WHEN YOU'VE HAD AN ACNE ATTACK OR EATEN GARLIC FOR LUNCH

Head over heels is a sexy position that's not face to face. Kneel down, cross your arms in front of you and lean forward so that your forearms rest on the ground and your derrière is in the air (cushion your arms on a pillow if you wish). Then rest your head on your arms. Your partner stands behind you and lifts your legs up by your knees until you're almost completely vertical, then he enters you from behind.

★★★

49

WHEN YOU HAVE PREMENSTRUAL SYNDROME

Studies have discovered two things: (1) boosted hormone levels means that right before your period is a high-octane time for you to make whoopee; and (2) an orgasm is a great cure for cramp. So, assume the position. Ask your lover to lie on his back on the bed and slowly squat onto his erect penis, facing his feet. Lean back as far as you can, being careful not to strain your lower back, and snuggle up against his chest. Reach back with your hands and caress his head. Your (bloated) tummy will look amazingly thin.

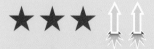

WHEN YOU'RE FEELING FAT

Try a classic pose to make you look (and feel) sexy and **voluptuous**. Make love in a side-to-side position, propped up on your elbow with the knee of your top leg resting on the bed. To your lover, your waist will look tiny and your hips will seem ultra-curvy.

WHEN YOU'RE IN A SINGLE BED

Start in the **missionary position** (see tip 1) and, with your legs and arms wrapped around him, gently roll over to one side. If there's too much weight on your bottom leg, you can carefully slip your legs between his.

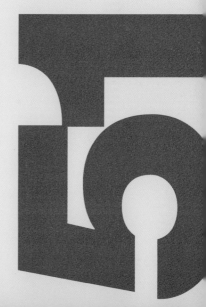

3

Intimate Sex

Even the most vertically-challenged relationship can get stuck in the middle of orgasmic nowhere after a while. Not to worry. All you need to get your return ticket to Ecstasy-ville are a few smooth moves. Slip any of the following into your next lovefest and let the pleasure ride begin!

SPICE IT UP

To get things sizzling again, here are some new positions for old lovers that are guaranteed to get the sparks flying.

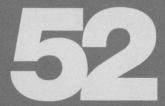

THE TWISTER

Your partner lies on his back with his legs spread slightly and his head propped up with a pillow. Start by lying on your back next to him, then swing your legs over his body crosswise and keep them close together so your legs are positioned perpendicular to his. Sit on his lap and lean back on your arms for support. Open your legs slightly as he enters you and begin making slow, swivelling, **corkscrew motions**.

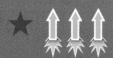

THE LEG LIFT

Your guy sits on the floor, his palms on the ground behind him and his fingers pointing away from him. His legs are splayed open and his knees are slightly bent. Placing your hands on the floor for support, you face him and straddle his lap. Raise your legs so your right leg rests on his left shoulder and your left leg is on his right shoulder. Keep your bodies close together so he doesn't slip out. The angle of his dangle will bring on deep **G-spot orgasms**.

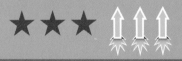

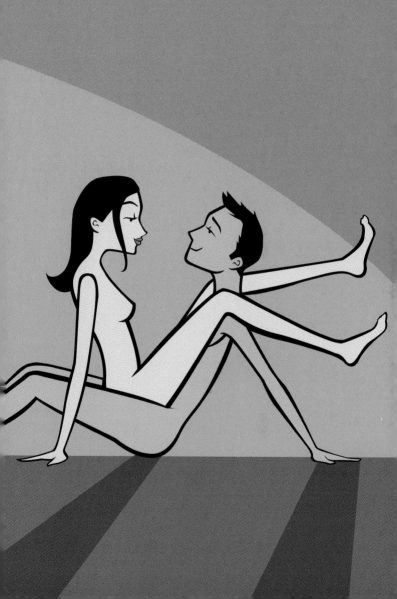

54

THE BONDER

You and your guy lie on your sides, facing each other. Now lean in and **scissor** your legs together. While thrusting, hold on close to each other for leverage and to create super-close friction. Rather than typical in-and-out thrusting, this sexual scissoring lets you and your guy please each other with grinding, circular motions.

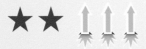

55 Aim to try out **ten new positions** a month (check out the rest of this book for ideas).

BODY BOOGIE

Physically, not all lovers are perfect matches. Here's how to mesh your bodies in the throes of love.

WHEN YOU'RE TALLER THAN HIM

He sits on the floor with his arms stretched out behind him for support and his legs crossed loosely. You climb onto his lap so you're straddling him in a kneeling position. Hold onto his shoulders as you lower yourself onto his erect penis, Keep your bodies extremely close together as **you take control** of the timing and speed of the thrusting.

WHEN HE'S A LOT TALLER THAN YOU

Sitting on top of him (see tip 2) ensures your love organs **stay connected**.

58

WHEN HE HAS A LAGER GUT
OR YOU'RE HEAVIER THAN HIM

A side move will let you work around your
bulges. Lie on your back with your man to
your right. He lies on his left-hand side. Bend
and lift your right leg up. Your man arranges
his right leg over your left and inserting his penis
in this position allows a nice leisurely pace. Crank
up the pleasure factor by grinding your buttocks
tantalizingly **against his pelvis**.

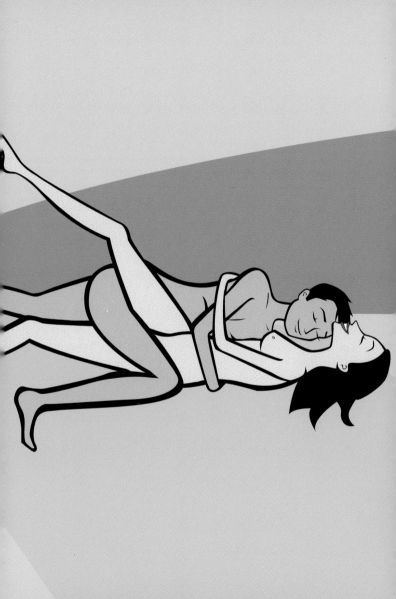

WHEN HE PACKS A BIG ONE!

If your man has a **large penis**, lying flat on top of him with your legs in between his and squeezing your thighs tightly together lets you control how deeply he penetrates you, while making sure his penis still gets fully massaged.

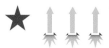

WHEN HIS PENIS IS PUNY

The **size** of a penis has very little to do with satisfying a woman. All it takes is 4–5 centimetres (1¹/₂–2 inches) to reach the super-sensitive nerve endings in your vagina. And nearly every penis, no mater how tiny when flaccid, is between 12.5 and 17.5 centimetres (5 and 7 inches) when erect. But you can still make it easier for him – and for you – by opting for a rear-entry position (see tip 5), which will make the most of what he has. Being on top (see tip 2) will also 'shorten' your vagina.

60

PUTTING IN THE PACES

According to studies, it's not the size of his package that counts – it's what you both do with it once it's in you that's the real key to how loud you'll be screaming with joy …

Allow him to penetrate you **more deeply**. Place pillows under your hips so your entire body is on an incline with your crotch angled up in the air.

When you're underneath, **clench your buttocks**. You'll lift your pelvis a little way off the bed and increase the blood flow to your pelvic area, making orgasm easier.

More thrusting does not necessarily mean more fun! Instead, get your man to rock your world by **rocking back and forth**.

The most **sensitive nerve endings** are near the opening of the vagina and in the head of the penis. So bring on a Big O by keeping penetration shallow.

65

After you've come and your vagina has **tightened** but your contractions are still going, ask him to keep on stroking inside your vagina until they stop. He should then quickly move to your clitoris and massage it. On the point of no return, ask him to put his fingers inside you again. Get ready to dissolve with pleasure!

To give him a rest while keeping him hot, ask him to **stop** while you do all the thrusting.

66

ORGASMS IN 0 to SEXTY

Here are some hurrying-up helpers for when you're having sex against the clock!

Do it in the morning! You're already horizontal, you have less clothes on to worry about, his testosterone level is highest, and you'll be in a carefree, glowing mood for the rest of the day.

67

68

Dress for speed: wear easy-to-unzip trousers (him) and a skirt with no underwear and definitely no tights (you).

When giving each other some simultaneous mouth sex, **keep pace together** by putting on some music with a strong, steady beat (pretty much anything from the 1970s will do).

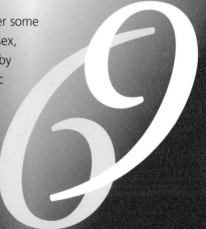

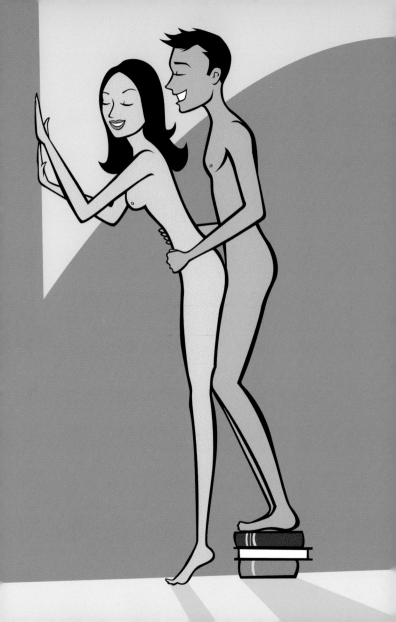

Rear entry is best from a standing
position if space is tight, but it can be
tricky to match
up your love organs
if you and your man
are different heights. For
guaranteed satisfaction,
face away from him and
bend over so that your
hands are flat on the floor and your weight
is forward (or just lean against a wall).

70

4

Daring Sex

Push your acts of amour to the utmost limit. Buckle up and get ready for an action-packed ride! Here, anything goes … but proceed at your own risk – you could find yourself in a whole new position, like court!

MARATHON MOMENTS

Try some of the following moves to make your carnal connection last from here to eternity …

Use a water-based **lubricant** like KY Jelly to increase the length of time you're able to have sex without risk of soreness.

Leaning away from each other is the perfect beginning for a **lovemaking epic**, although it probably won't give either of you a pulse-pumping orgasm. Start off by sitting on top of your man, facing him. Both of you then fall back in opposite directions supporting your weight on your elbows or hands, or you can lie flat on your back (whatever makes you happy). He gently thrusts from below for as long as your hearts desire (or his penis holds out), whichever comes first!

★ ★

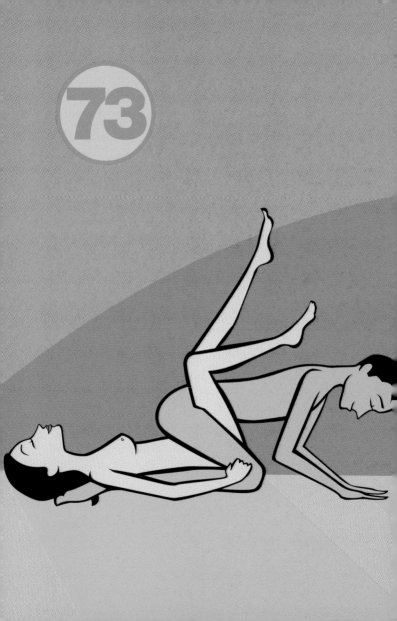

Do the chain. Lie back with your legs up, open and wide apart while your lover lowers himself on you face down, with his head by your feet and his legs over your hips so that his feet are on either side of your shoulders. You can rest your legs on his back and play with his balls as he thrusts backwards. For a real joygasmic thrill, hold on to his hips and pull yourself up in the middle of your love play to give your insides – and his penis – a total massage.

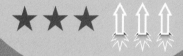

STAY IN CONTROL

Daring sex doesn't mean taking stupid risks. Make your contraception work for you and enjoy the double thrill of being sassy and sexy.

BE SAFE

The best position for sex is a safe one. Condoms are your best protection from AIDS, chlamydia and most other sexually transmitted diseases (STDs).

THE PILL

By suppressing ovulation, the Pill can lower your levels of testosterone. As a result, some women may feel a dip in desire. Any rear entry position (see tip 5) gives him access to play with your clitoris as he thrusts to re-rev your cravings.

INTRAUTERINE DEVICE (IUD)

The IUD can sometimes make sex a bit dry, which can be uncomfortable. Keep things sweet and sexy by using a side-entry position where your legs are interlocked. (He has one leg on the bottom, your lower leg comes next, then his top leg, then yours). Get him to grab your backside and hold you close to keep things tight and tantalizing.

DIAPHRAGM

Depending on the fit, this barrier device may hinder access to the area that requires stimulation. Sitting on top and leaning back so that your ankles rest on his shoulders will fully open your vagina and make sure his penis doesn't miss this hot spot during intercourse.

CERVICAL CAP

This device gives him free access to your vagina, so make good use of it! Have him come at you from behind, then rotate your hips in small, circular movements to ensure his penis bumps every part of your vaginal canal.

MALE CONDOM

Some men report reduced sensations from condoms, so really up his pleasure by sitting on top of him and leaning back and forth during sex to literally massage his penis with your vagina.

FEMALE CONDOM

Some women find that the ring on the base of the female condom stimulates their clitoris during sex. Make sure of this by using a man-on-top position with him riding slightly high on you (see tip 6/the CAT).

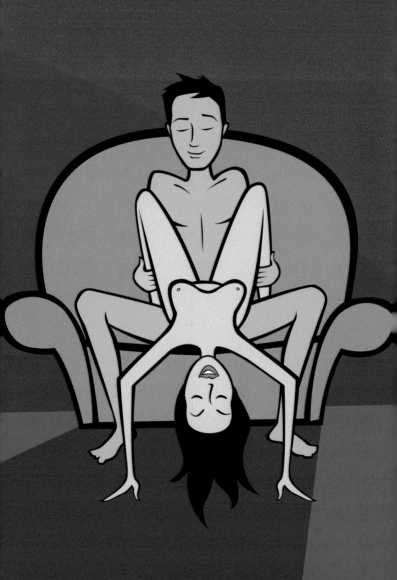

GET OUT OF BED!

Incredibly erotic hot spots for love trysts around the house will make you leap out of bed.

SOFA STRADDLER

Your partner **sits back on a sofa** (or comfy chair) as you straddle his lap with your legs splayed apart and your knees bent up against his chest. Then lean back so that you're almost upside-down, with your arms stretched behind you all the way to the floor to support your weight. Thrust back and forth, opening and closing your legs and clamping your PC muscles (see tip 27) around him. When you're ready for him to hit his passion peak, send him soaring by squeezing your PC muscles when he's completely inside you.

81

STAIR STOPPER

Kneel in front of your partner on the landing
of a staircase, with both of you facing the stairs.
While you reach up and hold onto each side of the
staircase for support (or to the stairs themselves),
he holds your hips and penetrates you from behind.
Be careful not to pull the banisters away!

 82

TABLE ROCKER

You **sit on a dresser** or table and he stands,
facing you. Now edge yourself down until he
can comfortably slip inside you. This body-rocking
move angles your vagina just right for a two-for-one
G-spot/clit climax.

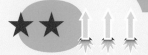

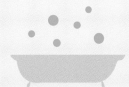

84

WATER PLAY

He gets in the **bath** first with his back to one end, his legs spread out in front of him and his knees slightly bent. (If your bath has taps at one end, make sure this is the way his back is facing.) Now you get in, sitting so you're facing him, with your arms propping you up from behind. Position your legs so they're bent on either side of him and your feet are resting lightly against the edge of the bath (if the bath isn't big enough to get a stable surface, just wrap your legs around his waist). Push your pelvis forward, lift your hips a little and use one hand to put him inside you.

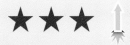

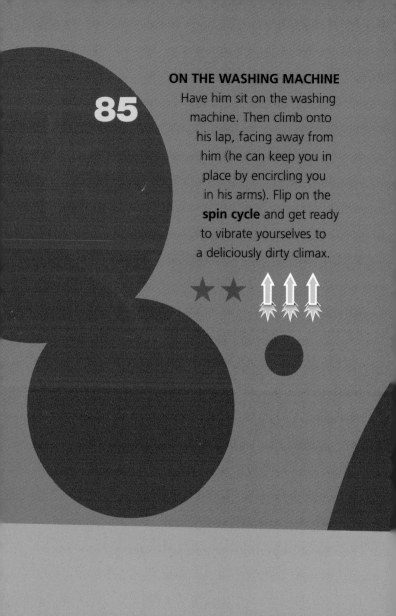

85

ON THE WASHING MACHINE

Have him sit on the washing machine. Then climb onto his lap, facing away from him (he can keep you in place by encircling you in his arms). Flip on the **spin cycle** and get ready to vibrate yourselves to a deliciously dirty climax.

★ ★

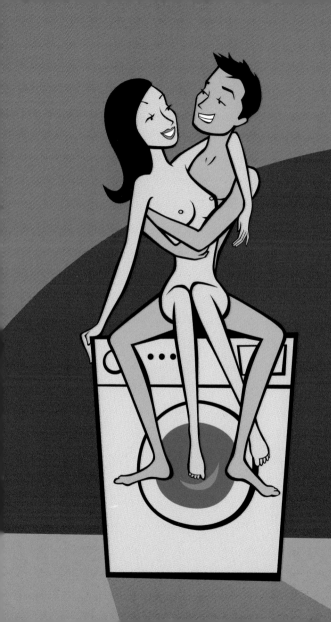

THE GREAT OUTDOORS

Whatever the scenery, the lack of a ceiling (and the risk of being spotted) will intensify the experience outside.

If you're going to have **sex outdoors** in any position other than standing, bring a soft blanket with you. Avoid using bug spray and sun block until afterwards – both taste awful!

ON THE BEACH

Making love on the beach can be a truly sexy. Use the **rhythm of the waves** to roll from underneath to on top and back again – you'll come oceans!

ON A PARK BENCH

Wear a long, floaty skirt **without underwear** and have him wear easy-access shorts. Keep things discreet by lifting your skirt, sitting on his lap side-saddle and wriggling gently until you achieve the desired effect.

ON THE GRASS

Relax on your stomach and elbows, and get your man to lie on top of you with his weight on his arms. Raise your hips slightly to increase penetration (and avoid ants in your pants!).

ON A CAR BONNET

Make sure the engine is cool and the car alarm is switched off! Then lie back with your hips at the edge of **the bonnet** and your legs spread wide. He stands between your legs, lifts them and penetrates you. Pull up to the bumper, baby!

IN A PARK

Stand facing a wall or tree with your feet about 45 centimetres (18 inches) apart. He stands behind you, bends his knees (unless you're taller than him) and enters you from below. If he wants to **show off**, he can hold your hips to steady himself and lean back, while you lean forward against the wall.

IN AN ALLEYWAY, FITTING ROOM OR OTHER NON-LIE-DOWN ZONE

He squats on his heels and **you sit**, facing him, on his upper thighs with your weight on your feet. Wrap your arms around him for balance. You'd better make this one a quickie!

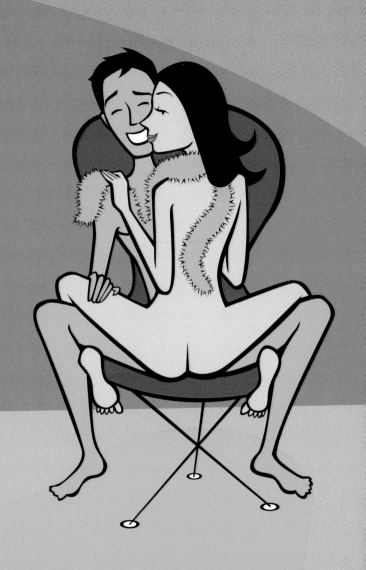

GO WILD

Rev up the raunch with some lurve tools and keep things sweet between the sheets.

There's nothing like **feathers to tickle** his fancy. Have a wide assortment handy – a feather duster, a boa, a quill, a peacock feather. Lightly brush over his whole love organ area while you sit on top of him (see tip 2). To really make him squirm with delight, concentrate on the spot where his penis meets his balls.

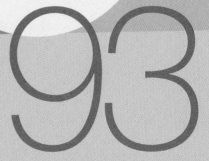

Give him a **lap dance**. Dress in crotchless panties and have your partner lean back on a strong, comfortable chair. Facing him and with your hands behind you resting on his knees, snuggle onto his lap. Lift your ankles up to rest on his shoulders. Start gyrating by inching yourself back and forth against his erect member. Slip him in and out of you to drive him wild with desire.

94

Put a small scoop of your favourite **ice scream** in your vagina, lie back and slip him inside you. Alternate with dripping warm – but not hot – wax over your bodies (be very careful, you don't want to cause third-degree burns!) to make your blood vessels dance with delight and give him a temperature-raising orgasm. Or try something bubbly like soda or champagne.

Have him **tie** your hands and feet together, then set you up on your elbows and knees. He then comes from behind to ravish you mercilessly while you love every minute of it.

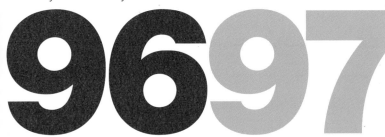

If you have **long hair**, climb on top of him (see tip 2) so you can seductively brush it back and forth across his body during sex.

Get fruity! A mashed banana or peaches inserted in your vagina is a delightful invitation for him to whoosh his penis around in it. Once you climax, switch to the 69 position for sweet afters.

Cool down your vagina with a **frozen-yoghurt** or flavoured-ice stick, then replace it with his penis. The heat of his organ against your icy skin will make it a sizzling sensation.

Wrap a **silk scarf** around your hand to stroke him. Rub it all over his body, tying it around his penis or testicles. Then use it to tie his hands or feet together and climb on top of him (see tip 2).

Get on the fast track to ecstasy! Lie back in the missionary position (see tip 1) and have him slip a **vibrator** against the base of your clitoris while he's inside you. He'll be able to feel the vibrations too and soon you'll both be pulsating with pleasure.

JOIN THE CLUB

To become a member, the only requirement
is body-blistering sex!

THE MILE-UNDER CLUB
Go scuba diving in warm
water so you can wear just
a bathing suit (this move also
works well in waist-high water).
Push the crotch of your bathing
suit aside, then wrap your legs
tightly around his waist (the water
will make you lighter than air).
Go with the flow, using the
motion of the water to rock
you up and down.

1

0

2

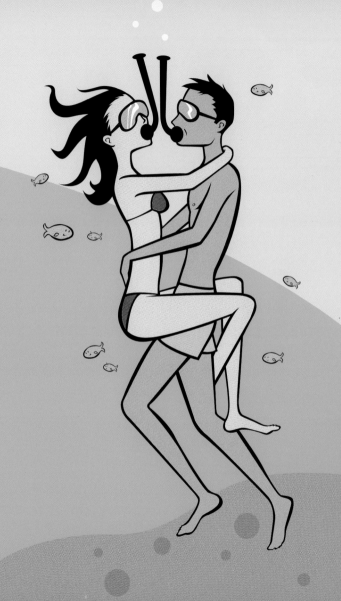

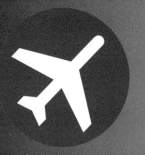

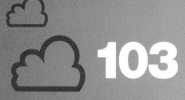

103

THE MILE-HIGH CLUB

Do it **on a plane** by sneaking off to the bathroom. Stand with your back to him and lean over the sink so he can swoop in from behind. Bonus: you can watch yourself in the mirror – this beats flying first class every time!

THE FAST-LANE CLUB

104

If you **get the hots** while driving your car, pull over in a secluded spot and jump on his lap. You can either face him with your knees pushed against your chest and your feet on the seat or hooked over the neck rest, or face away from him with your feet on the car floor. Either way, you won't be able to get much movement, so squeeze your thighs to increase the pressure on your love organs.

105

THE FAR-OUT CLUB

Doing it **in a boat** is like making love on a waterbed! But the position you choose isn't as important as how you position yourselves in the boat. Stand close to the centre of the boat and keep your body low. Motor boats and catamarans are the most stable, canoes the least. (Whatever you do, don't remove personal flotation devices and make sure you can both swim!)

5

Spiritual Sex

Your guide to nookie nirvana. Get ready
to have the best, most satisfying, intense,
mind-blowing sexual experience of your
life. But be warned – there's no such thing
as a spiritual quickie. Love made Eastern-
style can last for hours (read: hours of
pure soul-in-sync bliss … mmmm!).

SAY OHM-MY-GOD!

Prime your body for divine passion.

THE BRIDGE

Sit face to face with your legs wrapped around each other's backs. Slip him inside you and snuggle in by grasping each other's elbows, then lean back. Now see if you can tilt your head far enough back to rest it on the floor. Try to remain still and concentrate on your bodies, completely connecting the sexual energies flowing through you.

★★

106

THE JUMPING FROG

Start in the standard missionary position (see tip 1). He then rises up on **all fours**, and you raise your pelvis to meet his penis. As he stays stationary, start moving your hips up and down to get him jumping.

★★

107

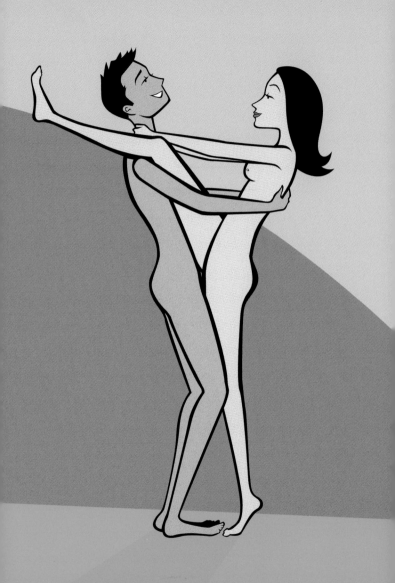

108

THE CRANE

Stand **facing your partner** with your left foot turned out, perpendicular to your sweetheart, and your right foot forward. His legs should be slightly bent, spaced about 1 metre (3 feet) apart. With your arms resting on his shoulders and his arms around your lower back, slowly pull your right leg up and prop your right foot on his shoulder. Once he penetrates you, ease into the vertical split by sliding your right calf as far up his shoulder as you comfortably can.

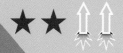

THE THREE-POINTED STAR

Lie **on your back** with your left leg extended straight up in the air and your right leg stretched out to your right on the floor, perpendicular to your body. Reach out across the floor with your right hand and clasp your right knee, forming a triangle with your right side, right leg and right arm. Your partner crouches at the bottom and enters you.

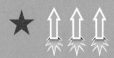

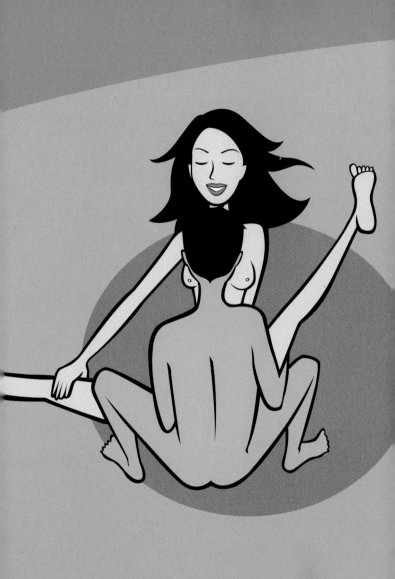

READ YOUR HOROSCOPE

Follow your zodiac to discover the most out-of-this-world position for you …

ARIES

An ultra-physical lover who like to take charge of her own sexuality.
Best Move: Anything on top (see tip 2) that lets you masturbate yourself to orgasm while controlling the thrusting.

TAURUS

A sensual lover who likes sex to last.
Best Move: A side-by-side position (see tip 4) that lets you do it just how you like it: in long, lazy bouts, with plenty of time out for kissing and caressing.

112

GEMINI

She likes variety, and lots of it!

Best Move: Start on top, so you're sitting straight up facing your lover. You can then lean forwards and backwards, or even swivel around to face his feet or roll over so you're underneath.

CANCER

113

A shy lover – she's never the aggressor.

Best Move: The classic missionary position (see tip 1) lets you feel like you're being seduced, especially if he holds your hands tight above your head.

LEO

She loves the foreplay almost even more than she enjoys the intercourse.

Best Move: Doing the 69 really lets you indulge your oral side.

114

115

VIRGO

Sexually mercurial, the Virgo lover likes to try many different things.

Best Move: Just about anything will spark your interest – and orgasms!

116

LIBRA

For her, it's all about the pursuit of pleasure …

Best Move: Rear entry (see tip 5), so you or your lover can caress your clitoris at the same time.

SCORPIO

Lusty and passionate, she likes to direct the action.

Best Move: Anything that puts you on top and in control of the depth and pace.

117

SAGITTARIUS

A strong lover, she enjoys strenuous intercourse and will make love through the night.

Best Move: Sitting on top and leaning back so you can see your lover as he massages your clitoris and breasts.

CAPRICORN

A straightforward and direct lover, she doesn't relish complicated sex.

Best move: The straightforward man-on-top move keeps things simple and sexy for you.

AQUARIUS

Curious and uninhibited, she likes to make love whenever – and wherever – the urge strikes.
Best Move: Usually standing and leaning over for a sexy quickie.

PISCES

An unusually creative lover who believes in the possibility of total ecstasy.
Best Move: You take classic poses just that little bit further. Lifting your legs over his shoulders while sitting on top of him, or sitting on his lap with your legs intertwined are two ways you might put your own stamp on making love (see tips 1–5 for more ideas).

ORGASMS
OVER
100
TRULY
EXPLOSIVE
TIPS

OOOOHH!

ORGASM TRAINING TIPS

According to sex pros Masters and Johnson, 10 per cent of women have never experienced the melting sensation of the Big O. But that doesn't mean they're ice queens. After all, orgasms aren't a basic instinct; they're a learned technique. Here are some sexercises that'll make you moan with delight:

1

Masturbation is the surest path to orgasm for both sexes – most people can bring themselves to ecstasy in four minutes flat. And research shows that the more orgasms you have by any means, the more orgasms you will have overall. Women who regularly let their fingers do the walking require less time to become aroused, have significantly more orgasms, greater sexual desire, higher self-esteem and greater marital and sexual satisfaction.

PRACTISE, PRACTISE, PRACTISE

2

Sex is like any other exercise. The more you do it, the better you become at it and the more you will enjoy it – the chemicals in your brain guarantee this. If you start making love more often, the chemical communication between brain cells quickens and intensifies because the impulses are travelling on a well-beaten path. The pay-off is more orgasms with less effort.

3

One fact that was probably left out of your biology class was the 'Use It' or 'Lose It' theory of sex.

Sexual abstinence in women causes what's known as **'vaginal atrophy'** – a general drying and closing-up of the vagina to the point where intercourse becomes virtually impossible. But studies have shown that women who stay sexually active, either with a partner or through self-stimulation, clock in more orgasms.

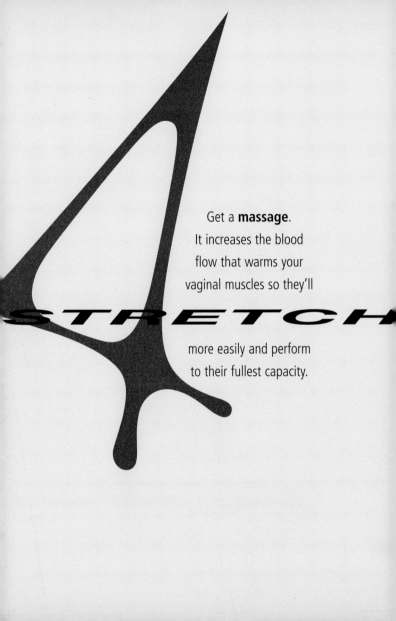

STRETCH

Get a **massage**. It increases the blood flow that warms your vaginal muscles so they'll more easily and perform to their fullest capacity.

Have what's known as an **active orgasm**. During intercourse, bear down, pushing the same muscles as though you are trying to expel something from your vagina. This helps you to push down against the penis or squeeze it up into you. **The result:** a longer and deeper orgasm. And it'll make his penis stand up and pay attention as well!

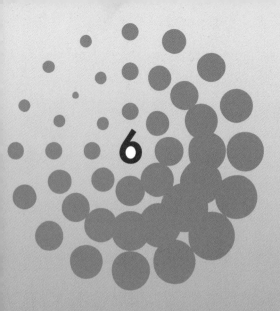

6

Buff **pelvic floor muscles** (the ones you clench when you're desperate for a pee) mean bigger, more intense and just plain **more orgasms** for men and women. Another benefit: the clitoris rests on these muscles, so the exercises also strengthen the clitoris and lead to stronger sensations. Start by squeezing and releasing the muscles 15 times a day, twice each day. Don't hold the contraction; just squeeze and let go. You can do the exercise anywhere: while driving a car, watchingTV, during a meeting. (Just don't announce it to everybody, okay?) Gradually increase the number of squeezes until you're doing about 75, two times a day. (See tip 39 for how to use them during sex.)

7

Working out for around an hour before your sex play gets you hot in every sense of the word. Any kind of vigorous physical exercise helps stimulate the blood flow and boosts aerobic conditioning, which preps the body for a meltdown orgasm. Also, studies show that people who exercise at least three times a week are more in tune with their bodies and more likely to be **sexually responsive**.

SECTION TWO

OH!OH!OH!OH!

SENSORY ORGASMS

You have five built-in tools to help you achieve orgasm – here's how to use them:

8: TOUCHING

The reason why studies find that only 30 per cent of women orgasm during intercourse is because women really need stimulation to the clitoris. But this little magic button is not a minipenis. The best touch? It's one that moves around your love button rather than one that applies pressure directly onto it.

9: SEEING

Seeing: Use your **eyes** as well as your hands and mouth. Just at the moment of orgasm, look deep into each other's eyes. An Archives of Sexual Behaviour study found that the erotic image of your lover in the throes of pleasure is an incredible turn-on for both men and women. You can close your eyes and have an individual experience, but if you keep them open, it's a shared one.

10: TASTE

Chocolate is known to contain natural feel-good chemicals that can boost the sweetness of your orgasm. Smear each other with chocolate body paint and slowly lick it off.

11: SMELL

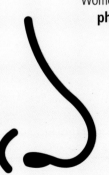

Women are more sensitive to **pheromones** – substances secreted by the body with an often undetectable odour that stimulates sexual desire. Nuzzling his armpit during orgasm can give you a heady whiff of his scent that'll make you swoon with bliss.

12: HEARING

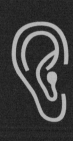

If you are going
through a lean period
orgasm-wise or just can't
seem to get yourself in the mood,
you might want to try role-playing.
This is not – repeat not – faking
orgasm. Role-playing is when you try to
cheer your orgasm into action when it
seems to be hovering just around the
corner. Exaggerate your movements and
sounds – wriggle, clench, moan. Now
throw in a few 'yes, baby, yes'
screams. The whole idea here is to
encourage your responsiveness
and cheerlead your orgasm
into action.

No-hands Orgasms

According to sex therapists, the best sex starts in the brain...

13 Think that you are enjoying yourself and you will. According to studies by Louisiana-based sex researcher Eileen Palace, PhD, when women learn to raise their expectations about sex, their bodies become more responsive within **30 seconds**.

14 In her research on easily-orgasmic women, Gina Ogden, PhD, found that 64 per cent had experienced orgasm through fantasy or dreams alone, **without any touch**.

15

A Journal of **Sex Research** study found 46 per cent of women and 38 per cent of men regularly indulge in erotic daydreams to keep their love juices flowing.

In fact, in some cases, fantasies made all the difference between experiencing an incredible climax or none at all.

16

Often the reasons for lacklustre orgasms have little to do with our bodies. Cutting out distractions like the phone, work stress and life worries helps you relax, and that helps to speed both your own and your partner's arousal along by widening the arteries of the vagina and penis so blood flows in freely to swell the tissues.

PHYSICAL
FOREPLAY

is an important part of a good sexual experience, but **mental foreplay** is equallly significant. Planning ahead makes your body far more responsive and primes it for orgasm.

18 Concentrate on your own feelings during sex

Women are so often concerned with pleasing their partners or worried about their failure to reach orgasm that they can't fully relax and go with their own flow.

19 Have an emotional orgasm

People think of sex as a very mechanical thing: How big?, how often?, how many times did I have an orgasm?, how long did it take? When we think of sex that way, something is lost — namely, the emotional component that bonds you and your man; the key to sweeter sex. When you catch yourself calculating — what should I do?, how hard? and for how long? — refocus your thoughts and try to concentrate on **how close you feel** to him.

The ultimate no-hands experience is known as the

extragenital orgasm (no vaginal contact). While 10 per

cent of women have this talent naturally, anyone can

develop sexy brain power – just replay your favourite

erotic images in your mind (if you need inspiration, flip

through a sexy magazine). Soon, you'll be able to

mentally bring on the Big O wherever you are.

Pleasure Timetable

The timing of a sexual encounter – the day of the month and even the hour of the day – can have a distinct impact on the quality of your orgasms.

21

The **Kinsey Institute** found that only 7.7 per cent of the women whose lovers spent 21 minutes or longer on foreplay failed to reach orgasm.

72

Synchronize your pleasure by giving each other a tongue bath at the same time. Lie head-to-toe and use your mouths as you would your love organs – imitate the grip of your vagina on his penis by contracting and sucking his tool. Meanwhile, he slides a firm tongue in and out of you. Get into a rhythm and then keep it up until you're both swallowed up in mutual ecstasy.

23

Do it **during your period**. The high levels of progesterone in your body will give you one of the raunchiest orgasms you've ever had. (It's also good for suppressing period pains!)

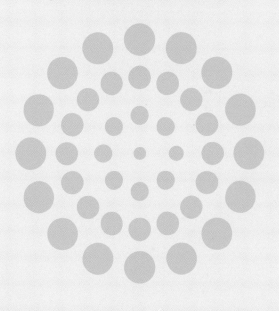

Right before **ovulation** and around the time you menstruate are two tidal waves of orgasmic energy... get a surfboard and have a fun ride.

Turn 30.

Studies from The Kinsey Institute show that compared to their twenties, when only 23 per cent of women regularly experience orgasm, by 30 around **90 per cent of them do**.

26 As strange as it may sound, many people tend to have sex at precisely the wrong time, physiologically speaking – at the end of the day when they're fatigued, stiff, full from dinner and so least likely to be able to be turned on orgasmically.

27

Testosterone levels are highest when we first wake up, and they decrease as the day progresses, which means your best orgasms are most likely to happen when you make love first thing in the morning.

28

Come first. In one survey of 805 nurses, the women who reported the least trouble in reaching orgasm were those whose partners had delayed their own orgasms until the women experienced theirs. The stop-start technique (every time he is close to orgasm, you stop stimulating him until he can regain control) is one way to slow him down.

DON'T STOP!

MOREGASMS

Or how to have as many moments of pure
bliss as you desire...

29

Women who regularly leap from one
orgasm to another report varied
stimulation is the key. Once
you've climaxed, simply
change the body part being
caressed or your lovemaking
position (and therefore the type
and location of stimulation).

Keep going.

The beauty of the clitoris is that it doesn't need to have any R&R (rest and relaxation) after climaxing. As long as it gets stimulation, you'll keep on coming. (One of the women who took part in a study had a staggering 134 moments of bliss in a row.)

30

A State University of New York Health Science Centre at Brooklyn study found that men can actually learn to climax and keep their erection through three to ten orgasms before exploding in the usual way. The key lies in helping him raise his orgasmic threshold by constantly approaching, then, just before he reaches the point of no return, backing away from ejaculation. Stimulate, then

31

stop and rest; stimulate, then stop and rest. According to the study, this helps men to separate the sensation of orgasm from the experience of ejaculation. And the physical result? He'll experience all the explosive feelings of orgasm without the ejaculation as often as he desires. And the emotional result? **He'll adore you forever**.

32

Have a **sequential orgasm**. This means a series of climaxes which come close together – anywhere from one to ten minutes apart – with a slight dip in your arousal in between. Oral sex followed by intercourse is all it takes.

THE ONE-HOUR
ORGASM

Six quick ways to have an endless orgasm...

33

Take a minute to do what you'd normally do in two seconds. Moving in slow motion makes you acutely aware of every sensation.

34

Leaning

away from each
other is perfect for
beginning a love-
making marathon. Sit
on top of your man, facing
him. Now both of you fall
back in opposite directions with
your weight on your elbows or
hands, or lie flat on your back
(whatever makes you happy). He can
gently thrust from below for as long as
your heart's desire (or his penis
holds out) – whichever comes first.

A simple sex surrogate
technique called **'vaginal
containment'** makes his
erection — and your
pleasure — last forever.
Straddle him or lie on top,
with his penis inside you.
He shouldn't move at all;
he just concentrates on
enjoying the sensation of
containment without the
extra rush of friction.

35

36

Hit the right nerves and sexual euphoria can reach new stratospheres. Research shows that the two genital nerves that surround the pelvic floor muscles give two kinds of erotic sensation. The first is a sharp twinge that occurs when the clitoris or base of the penis is erect and caressed; the second is a warm, melting feeling that happens when the inside of the vagina or the shaft of the penis is stimulated to climatic heights. Experience both types, one after another, in a single love fest, and you'll have what's called a blended orgasm, which can last for as long as an hour. One way is to stimulate one part of body – like the clitoris – until it feels too sensitive to touch, and then move on to the interior of the vagina until it feels aroused, and then return to the clitoris, and so on, and – sigh – on...

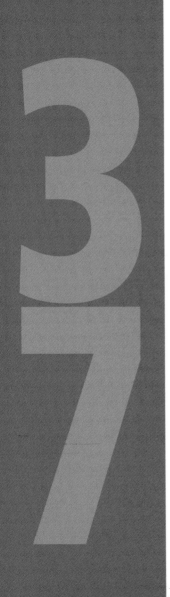

Recalibrate him. You can teach your man to last longer, plus give him a more explosive orgasm. While stroking his penis with your hand, ask him to rate his arousal on a scale of one to ten, with ten being orgasm. The idea here is to bring him to several peaks and then back down again without him climaxing. When he says he's reached a relatively low four, stop and tell him to breathe until his arousal subsides a hit. Now, rev him up to a heart-pounding eight, then stop until he's back down to a six or so. Finally, take him all the way. Later, he can work the technique into intercourse.

Tease yourself. Too many women try
to experience an orgasm as quickly as possible.
Instead, try prolonging your pleasure by
hovering at the brink of orgasm for as long
as possible by building up your arousal and
then getting your partner to shift his loving
attention to a less-stimulating part of your
body for a few minutes. The beauty of this
roller-coaster method is that arousal mounts
to such an intensity that when you finally
let yourself go, you're practically guaranteed
an outrageous orgasm.

NOW! ALL THE RIGHT MOVES...

Most women are well equipped to have an orgasm during intercourse. It's simply a matter of putting yourself in the best position to experience heaven....

39 **For a truly explosive orgasm,** squat on your partner (who is sitting up). Now thrust towards each other ten times. Stop and then squeeze powerfully with your pelvic floor muscles (see tip 6) ten times.

40 **Give** his and your love organs a massage in the middle of intercourse for a real orgasmic thrill. Lie back with your legs up, open and wide apart while he lowers himself on you face down, with his head by your feet and his legs over your hips so that his feet are on either side of your shoulders. Then hold onto his hips and pull yourself up a few inches. **Repeat until you collapse.**

41

Factor in the state of your mattress: The softer it is, the more the weight of you and your partner will push your pelvis down and make hitting the most sensitive parts of your vagina less likely. **For best results, try the floor instead.**

Studies have found that 77 per cent of women climax when they use the **coital alignment** technique (also known as the CAT). Your lover climbs on top, à la the Missionary, but instead of entering you straight on, he lies so his weight is totally on top of you and his pubic bone is actually rubbing against your clitoris. By settling into a gentle rocking rhythm, his penis rubs against your clitoris while moving in and out of your vagina.

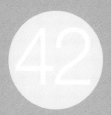

Three simple variations will up
your ecstasy odds exponentially
when using the Missionary position:

43

Your lover **raises his body**, resting his weight on his
elbows or his outstretched arms. This puts greater
pressure on your clitoris.

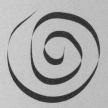

He puts his legs outside yours, while you keep yours together. This will give you lots of friction.

44

45

Raising your legs so that your knees are pressed to your chest and your legs are draped over his shoulders will make your vagina longer, allowing him to penetrate you more deeply. This will give you more friction and pressure exactly where you crave it most of all – your vaginal lips and clitoris.

46

The ultimate hot-spot position: place two stacks of firm towels together to form two sets of comfortable piles a few feet apart. Now face each other so that your backs are against the pillows. Arrange your bodies so one partner's legs are wrapped around the other's and your genitals easily connect. This position will stimulate multiple erogenous zones for both of you. You can vary the sensation if he pulls all the way out on some strokes and rubs his penis against your clitoris before thrusting in again. And the other advantage of this position? Four hands free!

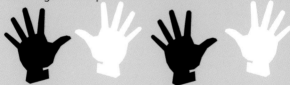

SATISFACTION GUARANTEED

These tips promise to please:

At something like 2,000 cycles per minute, the vibrator will send you both so high, you'll need clearance to land. If you don't have access to a sex shop, cheat by getting a battery-powered massager from the chemist. Don't worry about the shape — researchers have found it's the vibrations, not the shape, that triggers orgasm. Place it against your skin near the clitoris (but not directly on it, which can be too painful and intense).

48

Making love on a dryer during the spin cycle has a similar effect to using a vibrator.

If he tends to come before you and then immediately drops off to sleep, try the **Dual-Stimulation Technique**. Select an intercourse position in which your partner (or you) can easily reach your clitoris (such as the rear entry). This extra bit of stimulation may be all that you need to send you straight to heaven and back.

49

Lay back and do ... nothing. NOT trying for an orgasm is the surest way to have one.

50

51

After you've **climaxed**, your vagina will tighten up and then contract. If your lover alternates stroking the inside of your vagina with your clitoris, you'll keep on feeling the contractions every five seconds or so until you're completely taken over by delicious waves of pleasure.

52

Get stressed out. Conventional wisdom says that anxiety keeps us from climaxing. Yet there is also evidence to demonstrate that anxiety can increase sexual arousal by wonderfully concentrating the mind – in the same way that pre-curtain butterflies improves an actor's performance.

53

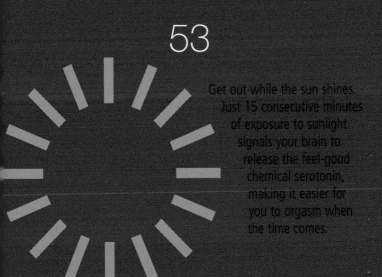

Get out while the sun shines. Just 15 consecutive minutes of exposure to sunlight signals your brain to release the feel-good chemical serotonin, making it easier for you to orgasm when the time comes.

Take charge of
your *pleasure*

We often think of an orgasm
as something which happens to us. Yet all it takes is
a little know-how to control of your own pleasure...

54

You can programme yourself to have a **coital orgasm**
(ie, through intercourse as opposed to clitoral
stimulation) using the Bridge technique. Your partner
(or you) touches your clitoris while he is moving in and
out of you. At the point of your climax, you stop
stimulating and concentrate on the rhythm of his
strokes as you orgasm. Each time you have sex, stop
stimulating your clitoris a little earlier: the penetration
will become the trigger for your mental Big O.

One technique sex therapists recommend to heighten intensity is to hover at the brink of orgasm for as long as possible. Orgasm is really just the release of extreme body tension. So the more tension you have in your body, the more pleasurable the release will be. Savour the bliss of being almost, but not quite there by backing off as you both get close to the Big O. Move to a less-sensitive area for a few minutes, then build the excitement back up again. You can increase and decrease your arousal a few times before surrendering to a head-to-toe burst of pure pleasure.

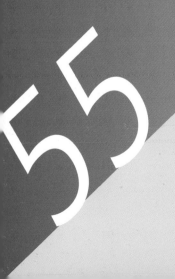

55

56 Clenching your buttocks

and your upper thigh muscles helps increase blood flow to your entire pelvic area.

This increased blood flow translates into greater vaginal lubrication and clitoral engorgement, which is believed to push the nerve receptors closer to the vaginal wall for greater sensation.

Just be sure not to hold your breath as you squeeze your behind – it oxygenates the muscles, making your contractions more efficient.

57

Anything that presses down on part of your lower abdomen during intercourse (his hand, your hand or squeezing the muscles or even doing a mini sit-up) massages your inner clitoris (see tip 71), putting you over the orgasmic edge.

YES!YES!YES!

58

Breathless orgasms... In the heat of passion, how you breathe is probably the last thing you probably want to be thinking about. But, surprisingly, changing your breathing pattern can help increase an orgasm's impact. The **faster** you breathe, the more **excited** you get.

Training the diaphragm, the muscular partition that separates the chest and abdominal cavity, can really increase the intensity of your orgasm. Practise puffing out through your mouth, huff-huff-huff-huff, concentrating on bringing each out-breath up from your belly, so you feel your diaphragm contracting to force the air out. Then during sex, as you feel an orgasm approach, try breathing more strongly and consciously than usual to force each breath out from your diaphragm. You'll increase the tension through your whole abdomen and upper body, raising the intensity of your ecstasy.

59

60

Position yourself so that your head is hanging off the end of the bed. This increases blood flow to your head and changes your breathing pattern, mounting the feelings of sexual tension and arousal.

61

Breathing through your nose is good for de-stressing yourself, but for truly great sex you need to breathe deeply through your mouth.

62 Deep breathing from the stomach instead of the chest during sex will relax you and increase the flow of sexual energy around your body. When you breathe in, push your stomach in as flat as it will go. As you release, push out and hold to the count of five. This makes you feel more energetic, increases your sensitivity to sex and slows down your reactions so you can really take pleasure in them.

Sex therapists advise women who have trouble reaching orgasm to change their breathing patterns. (If you hold your breath, exhale and vice versa.)

63

64

MOUTHWATERING ORGASMS...

Turn your orgasms into a delicious sexperience.

Try teaching him the Zen principle of oral pleasure: You can't 'see' pleasure in a woman, but you can feel it. With this in mind, he should place his tongue flat against your clitoris – the more it pulses, the hotter you are.

65

Remind him that his **tongue** is not a mini version of his penis. He should keep it soft and flat, and think of licking an ice-cream cone rather than plunging it in and out like a hydraulic drill.

66 The average woman needs her lover to spend about 20 minutes 'downtown' in order to make her body salsa.

67

instead of licking, hum – you'll both

experience orgasms that will make you

vibrate with pleasure!

68 Join your hand and mouth together to hold his penis. Move them up and down in a slow and steady rhythm. This is seriously orgasmic – it will feel like a hot vagina with magic fingers.

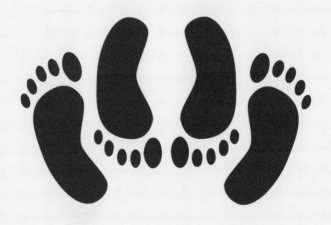

69 Make his entire body curl with pleasure by cradling his penis between your breasts as you lick him.

70 Most men prefer you underneath, like an oral Missionary position. One professional trick is to lie with your head thrown back over the edge of the bed to make your throat form one long, erotic passage.

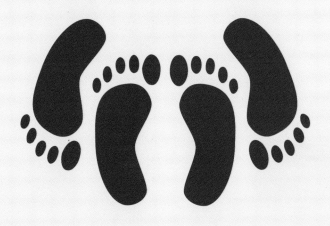

71 Find a rhythm during oral sex. Being in tune with each other's body signals – following breathing patterns, body movements and hip gyrations – will all help to keep you on orgasmic track.

ON-THE-SPOT BLISS

YOU

72 Rather than just a mini-knob of flesh, research published in the Journal of Urology confirms that the clitoris is also composed of around 23 cm (9 in) of highly sensitive erectile tissue that extends along the belly side of the vaginal wall. When stimulated in the right way, this inner clitoris can set off melt-down orgasms.

Best Move: Straddle him and lean back to push his penis against the front wall of your vagina.

The urethra, the tiny area of tissue below the clitoris that you pee from, is actually a sexual pleasure point. **Best Move:** The urethra is a good place to shift his tongue or mouth after you've had an orgasm and your clitoris is feeling too sensitive for continued direct stimulation.

73

74 Achieve maximum pleasure by having him stimulate all three parts of what is called the orgasmic crescent – a curved area that extends from the clitoral tip across the urethral opening (see 73 tip) to the G-spot (see 75 tip).

Best Move: Using tongue, hands or both, your lover should touch both the clitoral tip and the U-spot, while simultaneously pressing the G-spot.

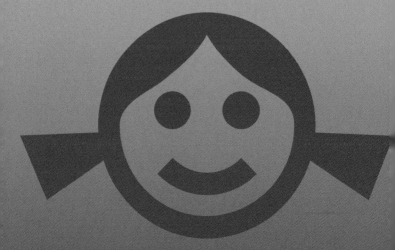

75

The G-spot is a sensitive mass of tissue one-third of the way up the front wall of the vagina (it feels like a soft marshmallow when touched). When pressed, it sets off an orgasm that is deeper and more of a full pelvic wave compared to the quick succession of mini-explosions from a clitoral orgasm. **Best Move:** Kneel at the edge of the bed, with your lover standing and entering you from behind.

According to a study published in the Journal of Sex Research, **the cervix** and the clitoris may be part of the same nerve network, which explains why, for roughly half of all women, stimulation of the cervix can lead to an intense orgasm.

Best Move: Try sitting on top of your partner while facing his feet for the deepest penetration.

76

77

The Anterior Fornix Erogenous is on the front wall of the vagina, about one-third of the way down from the G-spot. Research affirms that regularly pressing the area increased overall orgasmic response in the women surveyed, producing more intense – and simply more – climaxes.
Best Move: Lie face-up or sit on the end of the bed while your lover stands between your legs.

78

The cul-de-sac, found near the cervix, can raise your crescendo of bliss. Once you're aroused, it can be tickled by his penis and the muscles around your uterus will lift up.
Best Move: Make love in the Missionary position. Lift your legs up and back toward your body, sucking your stomach in.

HIM

79 Stroking his frenulum – the vertical ridge that extends from the tip to the shaft of the penis – will hit his climax switch. Not only are there more nerve endings there, but the skin is also extremely thin.

Best Move: Clenching your pelvic muscles just as he pulls out will give his F-spot a massage.

Many men are quite

surprised to discover

the range and depth

of the **sensation**

when you stroke

their raphe – the visible

line along the centre of

the scrotum. They

may even end up

ejaculating sooner

than they (and you)

originally planned.

Best Move: Excite

the raphe by gently

running your

fingertips

along it.

81

A man's **erection** doesn't end at the base of the penis. There's a railroad junction full of nerves in the perineum — that smooth triangle of flesh between the base of his penis and his anus which, when pressed, will send him straight into an orgasmic swoon.

Best Move: Gently rub the spot with the pad of your finger or thumb. (Pressing really hard with one forceful push can actually stop him from peaking, so be careful.)

82

Owing to its location at the base of the penis, a man's erection is more or less anchored upon the **prostrate** (also known as the male G-spot).

Best Move: Slip a well-lubricated finger through the rectum and probe the rounded back wall of the prostrate. When you start to feel a firm, rounded walnut-size lump, gently caress it while stroking his penis at the same time.

Both of YOU...

83 The anus is an often-missed hot spot, but it is crammed with sensitive nerves guaranteed to raise the orgasmic quotient.

Best Move: A well-lubricated finger gently slipped into the bottom just as climax hits.

84 Find your hidden hot spot. Make a fist and note where your middle finger hits your palm. Reflexologists believe stimulating this site, which corresponds with the heart centre, helps ignite your orgasm. Before sex, press the spot rhythmically with the thumb of your other hand for 15 seconds, then gently rotate the thumb there for 15 seconds. Repeat three times and then switch hands.

COSMIC SEX

How to achieve joygasmic nirvana:

85 He sits upright with his legs bent at the knees, but wide apart. You sit on top of him with your legs over his while you support his upper body. Now you both move in a rhythmic and slow fashion, while concentrating on deep breathing techniques. According to Taoists, this is the ultimate position to be in while the body orgasms.

Tantrics embrace each other's aura (energy fields said to buzz around each of us) for full-body orgasms. Start by imagining yourselves encircled in a glowing orb of light. Now, facing each other, he puts his Arrow of Love (figure it out) in your Seat of Pleasure as you lie back. Don't move: instead, just concentrate on breathing and looking into each other's eyes. Try to hold out for half an hour – the result will be heavenly.

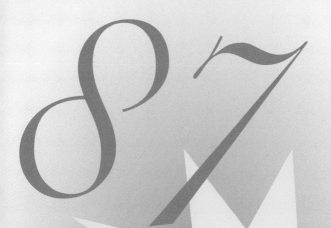

The Kama Sutra describes over 2,000 positions — all guaranteed to make you explode. Try the Mare, one of the easier moves. He sits, legs out, and hands behind him for support. You're on top, with your back to him, kneeling on either side of his legs.

60-SECOND CLIMAXES

Follow the next few tips and you'll climax before you finish reading this sentence...

88

The moves that work best .when you're in a hurry are generally carried out standing up, especially if space is tight. Unfortunately, the male and female physique rarely match up in a way that makes this feasible. Doing it on the stairs (with you one step higher) – or on an incline – evens things out. The same goes for bending over, with your bum towards his groin. In fact, anything done in the Rear Entry position gives the deep penetration often needed for quick sex and lets his penis hit the ultra-sensitive front of your vaginal wall.

89 Some women get an **overwhelming orgasm** *from quick intercourse without foreplay, but with deep penetration and they say that it feels different from the orgasms they get from clitoral stimulation or less vigorous intercourse. This sort of orgasm produces gasping, breath-holding, and a once-and-for-all climax. Too much foreplay de-rails this special response, which – when it happens – is as rapid as any man's.*

90

In one survey, which was conducted by Bowling Green State University, the majority of women polled reported that they preferred **'hard, driving sex'** to the 'slow, gentle' kind. Researchers concluded that since the vagina is most sensitive in its outer third part, women need to have constant pressure to orgasm during sex.

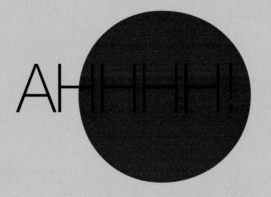

SECTION SIX

AHHHH!

ORGASM SECRETS

These little-known facts about your orgasms may be just the insider knowledge you need to up your pleasure quotient...

Rest up. When you're exhausted, you just don't have the stamina needed to achieve powerful orgasms.

91

If you're running dry, don't assume you're not interested. You can lubricate without being aroused, and vice versa. Lubrication is influenced by numerous outside factors – your menstrual cycle, whether you drink or smoke, medications like antihistamines and/or how much stress you're experiencing. The simplest solution is to add spit to the mix – yours or his – or water (see 94 tip). Otherwise, invest in a commercial lubricant (note for latex protection users: oil-based products destroy the latex) or condoms with extra lubrication.

93

Drink lots of **water** and skip the trip to the toilet before sex. Sex researcher Estelle Lauder, PhD, discovered that many women experience sharp, powerful orgasms as a result of the increased abdominal pressure of a full bladder.

94

Leave the other lubricants and gels in the bathroom cabinet (see 92 tip). Most commercial jellies can be too lubricating and kill the friction needed for orgasm to happen. Use **saliva** or water instead.

You've already heard all the boring stuff about the virtues of a balanced diet – but if you **eat right**, your libido functions better. In particular, stock up on anything containing vitamin B (vegetables, eggs, nuts, brown rice and fruit) and zinc (fish, liver, mushrooms, red meat and grains), all of which will enhance the efficiency of the nervous system and hence lead to better orgasms.

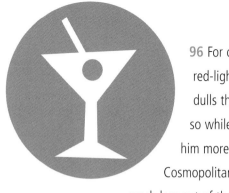

96 For orgasmic pursuits, red-light booze. **Alcohol** dulls the nervous system, so while you might want him more after three Cosmopolitans, you'll get much less out of the proceedings.

A half-glass **97** of **red wine**, on the other hand, will raise your testosterone levels and will make your reactions even more intense.

98 Speed things up with a double-sided approach. Sex researcher Shere Hite found that 70 per cent of women require clitoral stimulation in order to orgasm. So, combine a finger and a penis, a tongue and a finger, a vibrator and a tongue, then lay back and watch the explosions start!

99

Tobacco constricts the circulation of blood and may lower testosterone – the sex-drive hormone. Both of these are essential for an orgasm. A new study reveals that quitters had more orgasms afterwards than they did when they smoked.

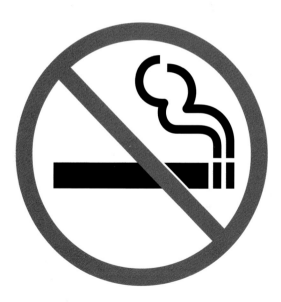

Drink a **coffee** with two sugars.

Since sugar and caffeine increase the heart rate

and give a surge of energy, they can make your

body more responsive to whatever nice things

may be happening to it.

101

Ginseng has been shown to add spice to your orgasms, but make sure you choose your root carefully. Some of the cheaper brands have been shown to contain less than 10 per cent of the potent plant.

102

Orgasms aren't a basic instinct that we're born with – they're a learned talent that comes with practice.

103

No two orgasms are alike for women. The climatic moment — supreme pleasure followed by a feeling of wellbeing and satisfaction — occurs in the brain's limbic system (or pleasure centre). **Sensations** can range from mild stimulation to an ecstasy so overwhelming that a woman momentarily loses consciousness. Recognize your range as opposed to going for an off-the-Richter Scale even, each and every time.

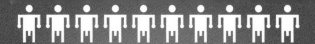

104

53% of men interviewed for The Janus Report

on Sexual Behaviour replied that their partner's

orgasmic pleasure was more important than their

own, compared to only **34%** of women.

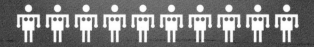

105

Between 10 per cent and 20 per cent of women have experienced a **sleep orgasm**. In that pleasurable experience, they are awakened by an erotic dream culminating in a climax. This is most likely to happen when you have been sexually deprived, but mentally stimulated. For example, he may be out of town, but not out of mind.

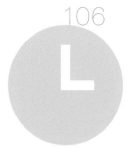

106

The average male
orgasm lasts for
10 to 30 seconds;
the average female one
is 13 to 51 seconds.

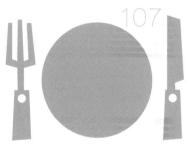

107

A rich meal eaten just
before making love
can inhibit orgasms.

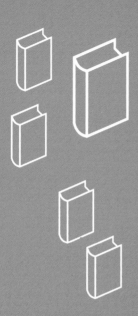

108

Study or get promoted.
One survey found that
the two best predictors
as to whether or not a
woman would be able
to reach orgasm during
sex were education and
social standing. Better-
educated women with
higher professional
status were more likely
to be orgasmic.

ORGASM BUSTS

Seven things can de-rail your pleasure.
Here's how to get back on track...

109

Problem: Breast-feeding – Prolactin, a hormone
that produces breast milk, dampens your sex drive.

Solution: Think about your baby. The hormone
oxytocin, which releases milk into the breasts, also
stimulates the contraction of the uterine muscles
and may help a woman to climax.

110

Problem: Stress
– Both cumulative and the daily, 'stuck in traffic' kind – can lower testosterone and DHEA, a hormone that enhances sex drive and acts as a mood-booster.

Solution: Before making love, take 20 minutes to re-group (take a walk, change into your playclothes or have a bath).

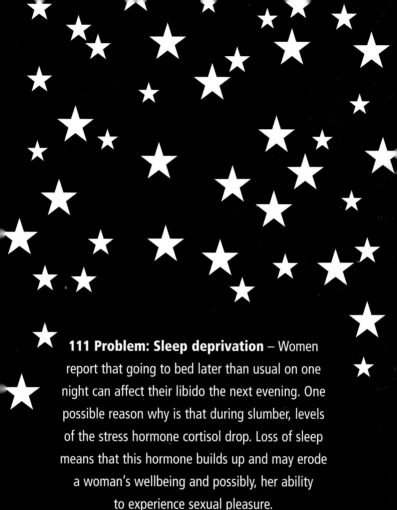

111 Problem: Sleep deprivation – Women report that going to bed later than usual on one night can affect their libido the next evening. One possible reason why is that during slumber, levels of the stress hormone cortisol drop. Loss of sleep means that this hormone builds up and may erode a woman's wellbeing and possibly, her ability to experience sexual pleasure.

Solution: Plan to get a full eight hours' sleep as soon as possible.

Problem: The Pill – By suppressing ovulation, the Pill can lower levels of testosterone and inhibit desire.

Solution: Work with your doctor to play with different levels of progesterone in your prescription.

Problem: The room in which you're making love is illuminated with 175-watt light bulbs.

Solution: Light some candles (but don't leave them unattended!)

114

Problem: You feel self-conscious about
your vaginal odour.

Solution: Don't douche. Arousal gives your vagina its
own natural muskiness. Look on it as your own custom-
made sex perfume. (If it's really unpleasant, though,
you may have picked up an infection and will need
to get it checked out by a doctor.)

Problem: You're scared you'll get pregnant or catch an STD (sexually-transmitted disease).
Solution: Always use a condom. (You should do, anyway!)

Problem: You've never had an orgasm.
Solution: Get a blood test. Your anorgasmia (lack of orgasm) may be caused by an injury or abnormal growth on the anterior pituary gland. Once the lesions are surgically removed, you'll soon become orgasmic.

QUICKIE SEX
OVER 100 TRULY EXPLOSIVE TIPS

Minute One:
On Your Mark

Let's face it, you're not always in the mood for some dreamy endless lovin'. Sometimes you're so damned hot you just want to fast forward past the Enya CD and the Tantric sex guidebooks and get on with the explosion.

The good news is that all it takes are five mad minutes to fire up your sex life big-time. That's right – 300 seconds. The fact is, there is nothing so exhilarating as fast, frenzied sex. Sex when you both have places to go, people to see, appointments to keep. Sex that is unplanned, impetuous and impulsive. Sex that borders on the forbidden or the foolhardy. Sex because you just have to have each other right here, right now.

Horny yet?
Then leave the dishes. Be late for work. And hold on to your hats – your sex drive is about to zoom from zero to 60 in less time than it takes to read this page.

7 REASONS TO DO IT RIGHT NOW

Having a quickie is essential for your mental health.

1

Stripped of all the trimmings, an orgasm is really just the physical release of built-up tension in the body. So quickies are a great way to de-stress (and much easier to get him to do than a massage).

2

Snagging a quickie is an instant mood lifter. Going fast and furious gets your blood flowing and boosts your endorphins for an oh-yeah booty bonus.

You jump-start your **inner sex goddess** by keeping your body pumped for action. According to research by Eileen Palace, PhD, the more stimulation your body receives, the more it is primed for being stimulated. So the more quickies you have, the more quickly you will get turned on.

A new way to spell relief: **Q-U-I-C-K-I-E**. According to research by Lawrence Robbins, MD, a dose of instant sex can help relieve women of pain from migraines (and it's a lot more energizing than a tranquillizer).

You're acting according to your biological nature. Humans were designed for fast sex, say evolutionary psychologists. The animal kingdom wasn't used to wasting time. The more time you spent copulating, the more vulnerable you were to being consumed by some woolly thing (and we don't mean your lover).

Quickies are efficient. They get the job done. So you get to have sex and still get a decent night's sleep at the end of it.

They're empowering. Yes, that's right. What could be more of a power trip than inciting your lover into a sexual frenzy?

4 REASONS HE WANTS YOU TO DO IT NOW

All it takes to plaster a goofy smile on his face is 5 minutes.

Men are suckers for a little mystery – studies show that the possibility of conquering the unknown is a top reason for why guys stray. Surprising him with some sex-on-the-run will stop him from thinking he knows all your secrets – keeping him as faithful as a St Bernard dog.

Research has found that an **occasional quickie** can be the answer to a lot of his sexual anxieties. There's no losing sleep over how long he has to last or whether he is giving you enough foreplay. All he has to do is get an erection and use it.

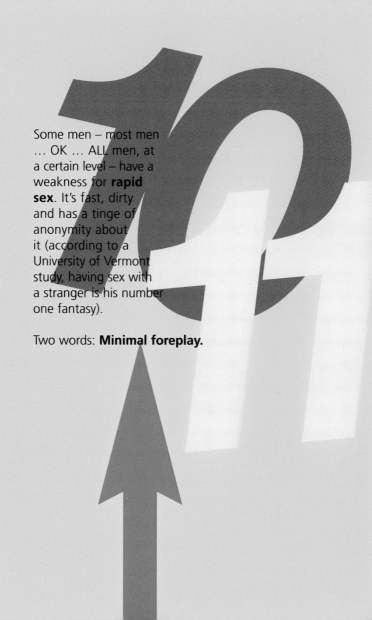

Some men – most men … OK … ALL men, at a certain level – have a weakness for **rapid sex**. It's fast, dirty and has a tinge of anonymity about it (according to a University of Vermont study, having sex with a stranger is his number one fantasy).

Two words: **Minimal foreplay.**

IF YOU'RE STILL NOT CONVINCED

7 MORE reasons why you really should do it now –
if only to have a more bonded union.

Who has the time or energy for all the prep work
that goes into prolonged sex? Dimming the lights to
a flattering glow, burning candles, bracing yourself
for the never-ending G-spot expedition … yawn.
Sex is like dining. Sure, the five-course gourmet
deal is delicious. But sometimes, nothing but a
hamburger will do.

Even a tired quickie can convey **more tenderness
and caring than long hours of lovemaking.** Bet
this sounds familiar: You're exhausted. He wants
sex. You love him so you don't want to reject him
and you know you can do just about anything for
five minutes (and chances are, once you get started,
you'll find tip 66 kicking in).

While quickies may not be able to save a relationship in nosedive, they're certainly the easiest – and fastest – way to **revive a boring sex life.** If you're used to a certain method of making love, a fast body bash can break a ho-hum routine (and it beats dressing up in that French maid's outfit any day).

You'll keep the flames burning. Passion doesn't automatically keep going – you've got to work at it, say relationship psychologists. The role of a quickie is to turn up the heat once in a while.

Quite simply, **your relationship depends on it.** According to a study by Ellen Bersheid, PhD, a psychologist who researches close relationships, in order for love to thrive, it's essential that lovers experience minor interruptions so that they can recapture an awareness of their emotional involvement. Because you've behaved unexpectedly and interrupted a pattern (that is, your usual Saturday night making-love-in-bed), he'll be reminded of how much he loves you.

17

Nano-second sex reminds both of you that no matter how crazy life gets, there's always a little window of time to connect as a couple. (Three quickies a week is only 15 minutes. Anyone has time for that.)

The after effects last a long, long time. One poll found that couples who regularly speed up sex, kiss, cuddle and hold hands more. How's that for afterplay!

18

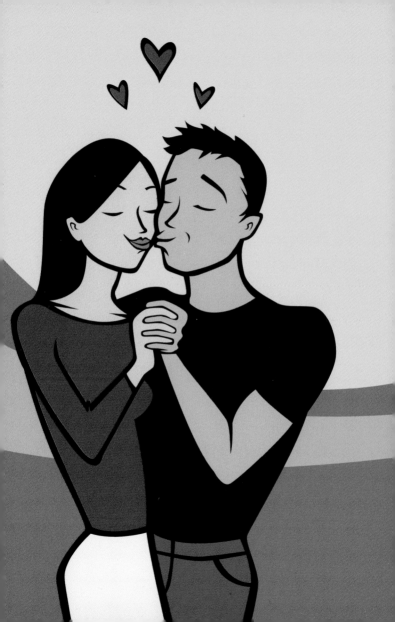

SO NOT TRUE

Take your time and read these quickie myths.

MYTH: Quickie sex bites.
TRUTH: Arousal is a mysterious and powerful thing, so the frantic abandon of a quick fix can ignite a climax that's every bit as explosive as a marathon session in the sack.

MYTH: Women need at least 72 hours of foreplay to have an orgasm.
TRUTH: Actually, cutting to the chase sexually can pay off passionately for both of you. The evidence shows that we don't exactly need a lot of time to experience sexual nirvana – according to studies by sex researchers Carol Darling, PhD, and Kenneth Davidson, women can, on average, reach orgasm in 8 minutes with a partner. In other words, full-blown, drawn-out foreplay, while tasty, is really just additional sauce.

MYTH: Women hate quickies.
TRUTH: *Au contraire*. In one survey conducted by Bowling Green State University, a group of men and women, aged between 25 and 43, were asked, 'If you had to make one choice – and you could have only one – which would you choose: hard, driving fast sex or slow, gentle sex?' The majority of the women wanted to get hammered.

MYTH: Languorous lovemaking, hours in bed, kisses and caresses that go on forever and back rubs are necessary for good sex.
TRUTH: You can be TOO relaxed. According to a Tulane University study, since orgasm is a tension release, the more STIRRED you are mentally during sex, the higher your bliss potential.

MYTH: If he wants a quickie, it means he doesn't love you.
TRUTH: Every act of sex doesn't have to be a relationship seminar. Studies show that couples who don't mind doing it quickly every once in a while have MORE sex because they don't place so much emphasis behind the meaning of each carnal moment together.

Minute Two:
Get Ready

True, the great thing about a quickie is that it's pretty much a no-frills, anything goes proposition. There's no obsessing about setting the perfect mood, wearing the right lingerie or putting on clean sheets. For that matter, who needs sheets at all?

But the reality is that sex never happens spontaneously. If you expect it to, you're setting yourself up for disappointment. Generally, there's always a prelude that leads us to be sexual, say sex experts. A certain loving touch, a special outfit that gets us in the mood. Bottom line: whatever our preliminaries, we never come cold to sex, we always prepare.

So here are a few fast-and-loose guiding principles to prep you for chasing the World's Fastest Orgasm title. What are you waiting for?

ONE MINUTE TO BETTER WHOA!

Learn to exercise control.

Limber your love muscles. According to the American Association of Sex Educators, Counsellors and Therapists, toning your pubococcygeus (PC) muscles helps lubricate and stimulate you, making your orgasms come on more quickly and more intensely (this goes for men, too).

- Find the right muscles – the ones you use to stop your urine flow.
- Exercise them – squeeze and hold tight for three seconds. Relax for three seconds, then repeat, building up until you can maintain a squeeze for ten seconds. The more you do, the stronger the results.

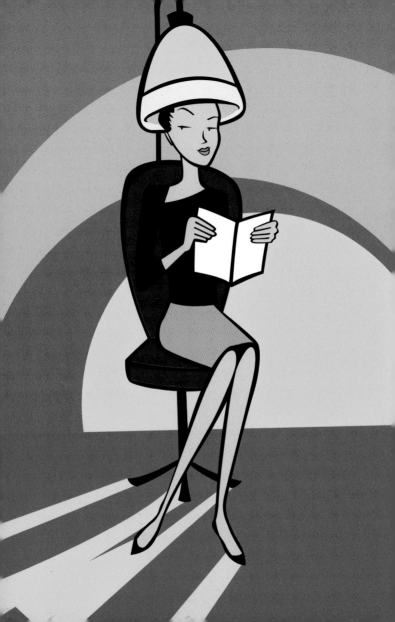

No one will know what you're doing, so go ahead and **squeeze when you're stuck in a traffic jam,** you're bored at work or getting your hair done.

Bonus: Squeezing those PC muscles makes you aware of your vagina and clitoris, sending little turn-on messages to your body so you end up effortlessly doing tip 64.

To use during sex, squeeze as he slides out and release as he plunges in. It'll feel like a suction cup around his penis and create tantalizing friction for both of you.

A-SEX-ORIZE

How to dress for the occasion.

Plan on staying semi-clothed. If you're prepared to get naked, you're not impatient enough to get into the swing of the quickie (unless you're planning tip 78). Of course, ripping your clothes off is a different story.

Wear a suspender (garter) belt to work, you naughty thing. It'll give him access for later and get you into tip 64. No tights (pantyhose) unless you have a run in a strategic spot.

Slip into something new. According to one survey, husbands who fail to notice that their wives changed their hair colour from black to blonde literally leapt to attention at the sight of a fresh-off-the-rack pair of lace underpants or an unfamiliar push-up bra.

You don't have time to **worry about your body during a quickie.** So disguise your jelly belly with big panties that cut just above the belly button and make your stomach look flatter, a more practical solution than sucking in your breath.

Forget fashion and **slip into a longish, loose skirt** – it's ideal for hiking up and making a quick discreet connection in public places.

If you can't skip knickers altogether, **make them edible** (see tip 36 for buying info).

33 34 35

A sexy teddy or leotard that opens at the crotch will have you ready in a snap.

Y-fronts or boxer shorts for him were designed with a quickie in mind.

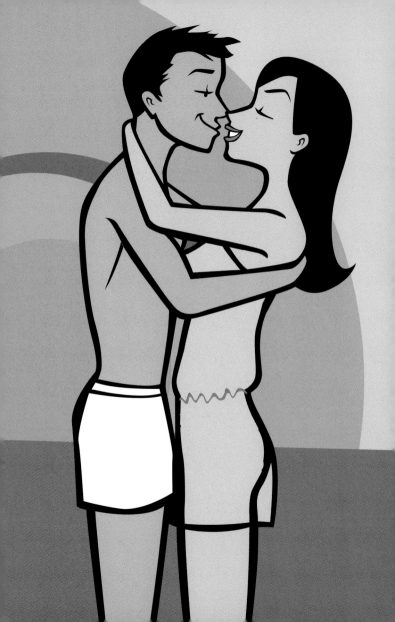

INTRODUCE A THIRD PARTY

There's nothing like your own personal joystick to get a buzz in a flash.

36

A Magic Wand vibrator, with a ball-shaped vibrating head, flexible neck and long cylindrical body is best for both of you (available on-line from www.annsummers.com).

37

Using a battery-operated vibrator will ensure that you don't run out of steam mid-play. According to the sex toy store Good Vibrations (www.goodvibes.com), the best are Japanese-made.

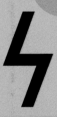

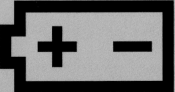

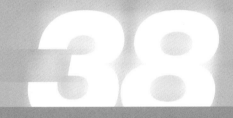

38

Best high-speed move: Press your new love toy against (not on) your clitoris or insert it into your vagina. Run it along the bottom side of the penis. Indirect vibes create a deeper, more satisfying orgasm than ones that hit your bulls-eye.

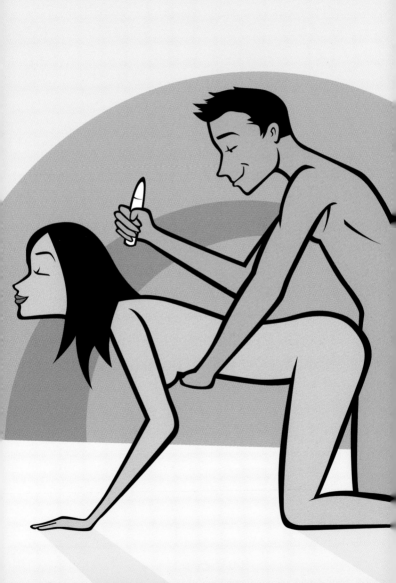

Woman-on-top and rear-entry positions allow plenty of room to get a good buzz going.

39

40

Pressing the head of the vibrator against your tummy will make you arch with ecstasy.

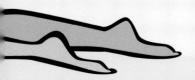

HURRY-UP HELPS

Tricks to heat the action up in a flash.

Eat right. Chocolate contains phenylethylamine, a mood-boosting chemical that can incite lust. Oysters are a good source of zinc, which studies show help his standing-to-attention powers. Other research suggests that seafood in general, which is high in protein, is also high in tyrosine, an amino acid that can act as a libido pick-you-up. And chilli peppers trigger the release of endorphins, feel-good brain chemicals that make you ready for action.

Get wet. Studies by sex researchers John Wincze, PhD, and Patricia Schriener-Engel, PhD, have shown our body's responses sometimes take time to catch up with our mental urges. Adding a drop of water-based lubricant to the head of the penis (or condom) before sex will keep your body and mind on the same sexy wavelength.

43

Forget crooners like Luther Vandross and Natalie Cole. A study from Loyola University discovered that heavy metal and other hard-rock variations get his pulses (and other bits) racing. So make sure you have a Limp Bizkit or Linkin Park CD in your collection.

Stick your schnoz in his underarm. A recent Bern University study found that this is where a whiff of someone's scent can send you into a sexual frenzy. A sniff of lavender and pumpkin pie will have the same stiffening effect on him – the Scent Smell & Taste Treatment and Research Foundation in Chicago discovered that these combined odours increase penile blood flow by 40 per cent.

44

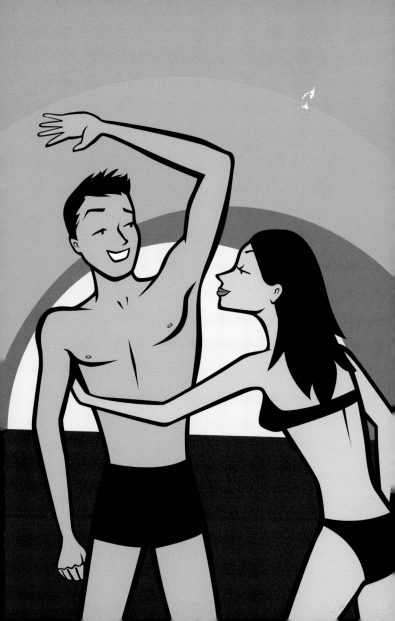

Come – er – prepared. Studies on **easily orgasmic women** (those who climax more than 90 per cent of the time) have found that they often anticipate steamy encounters hours – even days – before (see tip 64 for suggestions).

You knew there had to be a good reason you were logging all those hours in tush-tightening class. A University of Washington study found **a quick 20-minute workout primes our bodies for sex** (and not just because we're at the gym ogling sweaty, buff men doing bench presses). It seems a hard-pumping heart sends blood to all extremities – including sex organs. So pump your own iron before you pump his.

Bump up your secret hot spot. Build sexual tension with this indirect pleasure prep: massage the area about one middle finger length below your belly button. Pressing it gently for about three minutes helps promote blood flow, firing up the whole pelvic area.

Keep a naked snap of your man (or anything you think looks really sexy) in your wallet. You'll feel flirty all day.

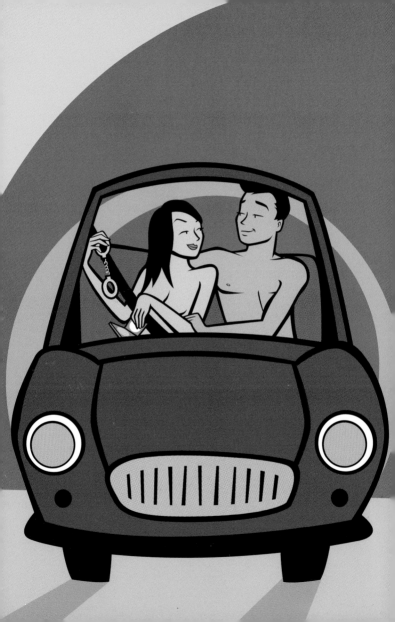

49

Carry a quickie kit:
Keep condoms, any props
like scarves or handcuffs
(for a little light bondage),
lubrication and a compact
mirror and hairbrush (for
post-sex sprucing) to hand,
so that in the midst of
passion, you don't get
stalled on technicalities.

PICK-YOU-UPPERS

Fuel up with the following to turn your libido into Speedy Gonzales.

50

According to studies, **fish and beans** can turn his wood from willow to mahogany.

51

Take a daily dose of libido-boosting **homeopathic remedies** like graphite, lycopodium or pulsatilla and say, 'Hubba-hubba'.

52

Red wine boosts testosterone levels to make your reactions raunchier – especially if you're on the Pill.

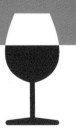

53

Give yourself an **energy boost.** Vitamin C energy powders will give you the orgasmic stamina you need for a quickie.

Get a buzz on with bee pollen. Research shows that it lifts energy levels, libido, sexual potency and fertility. How sweet it is!

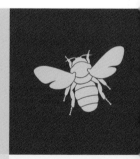

Spicy foods such as chillies, garlic and onions ignite sexual passion. Just make sure you carry breath mints with you!

HOT AND BOTHERED
Give him THAT sign.

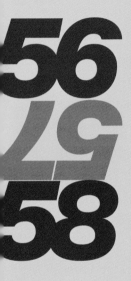

56 Simply take his fingers and **put them in your mouth**. It will send an instant message to his groin.

57 Get right to the point – lift up your top and **press your cleavage** against his back.

58 Try **blinking** in time to his breathing – it's like flashing the word SEX in front of his eyes.

Place his hands where you want them – on you.

Create a quickie code, perhaps a wink or a secret handshake that says in no uncertain terms **'You, me, here, now'**, to preclude any awkward misunderstandings or long, boring waits in the bathroom for an unwitting partner.

59
60
61

Stare directly at his **crotch.**

When you're out in a **public place,** disappear for a few minutes then, when you return, hand him your panties. Or whisper that you are wearing tip 33 in his ear.

Greet him naked.

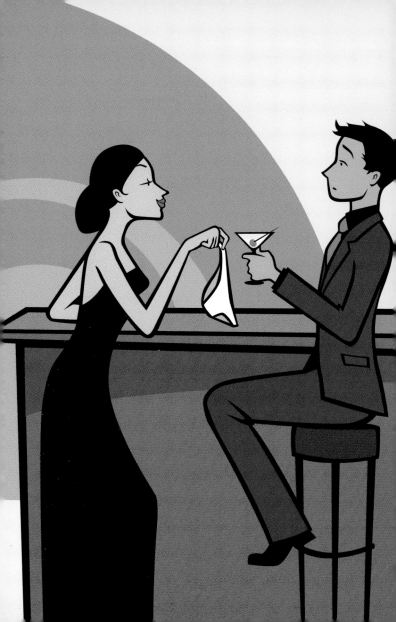

Minute Three:
Get Set

Here's a newsflash: he doesn't hold a patent on horniness. It seems that both men and women have a supply of the hormones that propel the sex drive into amorous action: oestrogen, progesterone and testosterone.

But there's more to keeping your sex drive in gear than pushing the right buttons or putting a tiger in your tank. To have all the heady force of a turbocharged engine in peak performance, your sex drive has to be revved emotionally as well as physically. That goes for men as well as women.

Here, then, is the owner's manual for getting your mind and body focused back to where it damn well should be – sex! Your car mechanic may not know about them, but these aids are a sure-fire guarantee for ignition.

MENTAL HURDLES

Having an orgasm is often 80 per cent mental and 20 per cent physical. Here's how to get in the right state of mind to enter the Oh! zone.

Sex up your brain. Fantasize or watch something sexy to get you in the mood (log on to www.nerve.com if you don't have any steamy video tapes to hand).

64

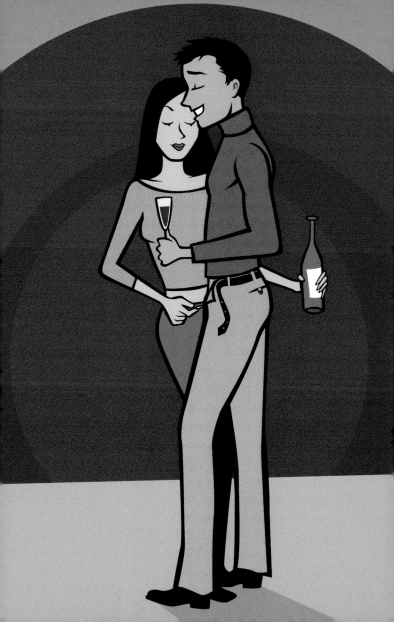

Have a few drinks. While studies show that booze inhibits men, it actually has the opposite effect on women (as long as you keep it to two).

Think you are enjoying yourself and you will. Even if it feels as if you're just going through the motions at first, it will feel great in just a minute. According to studies by sex researcher Eileen Palace, PhD, when women raise their expectations about sex (and think, 'of course my toes will curl'), their bodies become more responsive within 30 seconds.

Get over it. Sex doesn't cure cancer. It also doesn't ensure world peace or bring down superpowers. The point is, getting it right every time isn't that important. If you start fretting about whether you'll break sexual records, just start repeating to yourself: 'This feels good, this feels good' – in other words, forcing your mind to go with the flow of tip 66.

MASTER YOUR OWN DOMAIN

Give yourself a helping hand to remain in a sex-ready state.

When masturbating, women do not linger any longer than men: Kinsey reported that it takes an average of about three minutes for both to come to orgasm.

Studies have found that the **erotic highs** from masturbation can last a few hours. So you can speed things up by letting your fingers do the walking long before your lover arrives on the scene.

In one poll, 95 per cent of men said they like it when **their lover creates her own pleasure.** On one hand, it takes the pressure off them. On the other, it's just plain hot (if you really don't know why, see tip 95).

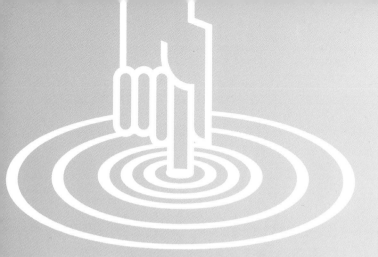

71

Wet your fingers first.

72

Locate the target: Touching the clitoris directly may be too intense, which means that instead of building up to an orgasm you may feel numbness or even pain. To avoid this, press your index and middle fingers on either side of outer lips, gently squeezing the fingers together in a circular motion to stimulate the clitoral ridge underneath.

73

Squeezing and contracting your thigh muscles while thrusting helps massage your clitoris against his hard body.

A QUICKIE FIX

Bed-tested techniques guaranteed to make the Earth move in sync.

You're Hot, He's Not: The quickest way to get a man hard is to go straight to the heart of the matter: his penis (a Pirelli calendar nearby doesn't hurt either). Three tips: use a firm grip, a wet hand and flick your tongue.

74

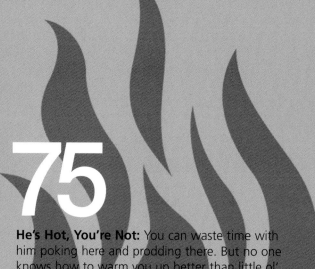

75

He's Hot, You're Not: You can waste time with him poking here and prodding there. But no one knows how to warm you up better than little ol' you. A little spit or lubrication on the finger will speed things along. Put your hand over his to make him putty in your hands (see tips 71 to 73 for beginner's help).

He Needs To Slow Down:
According to the Kinsey Institute clock, a man can go from start to finish in one minute. To pace himself to last another 120 seconds, he can:

- Flex his muscles (when a man contracts his PCs – direct his attention to tip 24 – he can lower arousal a few notches).
- Breathe deeply (it directs blood away from his penis).
- Open his legs (when he is lying on top, he can spread his legs to take the pressure off his testicles – when they are too compressed, they become overstimulated).
- Change gears (simply changing positions can halt his momentum).
- Take it out (it removes him from the seat of action – blowing warm air onto it will keep him hot without exciting him to the point of no return).

76

77

You Need To Speed Up:
Once a woman is hot, she can keep pace with any man. The trick is getting to the race on time:

- Begin without him (see tip 46).
- Let him help you get a head start with a one-minute visit south of the border (studies show oral sex has the double bonus of quickly lubricating and stimulating you in all the right places).
- Give yourself a helping hand (see tip 75).
- Position yourself correctly (getting on top will help his penis connect with your clitoris while rear entry is best suited for hands-on sex).

Minute Four:
Go!

With time at a premium, we're going to cut to the chase. Here, handy tips for doing the horizontal indoors, outdoors and everywhere in between.

Yes, it's risky. That's precisely the point. Moderate fear – not staring-down-an-agitated-lion fear but the kind you feel when you could potentially be caught doing something naughty – causes the production of adrenaline, the sexy pick-me-up you manufacture when you're aroused. But exercise discretion. While the other half of the thrill of a quickie is that the world, so to speak, is your mattress, you can be fined or arrested if caught.

GET YOUR TIMING RIGHT

When it comes to catching the orgasm express, timing is everything.

Skip lunch and have a nooner instead. Testosterone levels in adult males are subject to circadian rhythms, researchers have found, meaning that they rise and fall in 24-hour cycles – and they tend to peak shortly before 12 pm.

Your body starts screaming yes, yes, yes around mid-cycle (14 days after your last period) when oestrogen levels are at their highest.

Don't do it: **hold off having sex for two weeks** and it'll add instant heat to your flash-in-the-pan coupling.

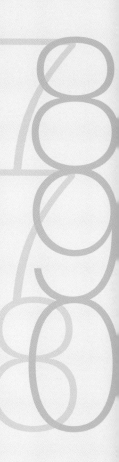

Make a quickie your wake-up call. It's better than an alarm and the chances are, he'll already be hard.

81

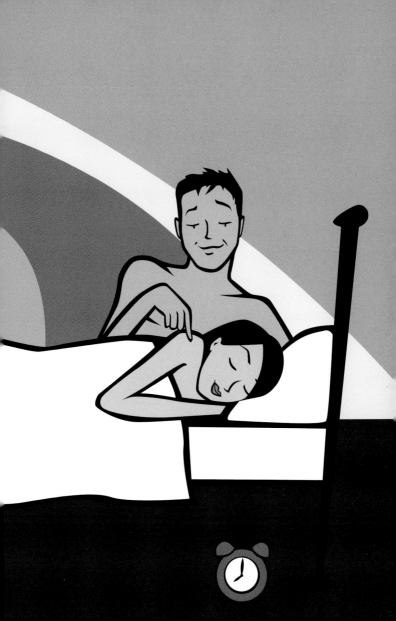

LOCATION, LOCATION, LOCATION
Any where, any time, any place.

Concrete Jungle
Unless you're a masochist, if you're romping in an alley or on a road, you'll want minimal ground contact
- For a raunchy position that stops your clothes from getting dirty and your bottom getting cold, he should **squat on his heels while you sit on his upper thighs facing him** with your weight on your feet. Wrap your arms around him for balance.
- Another hot move: Stand facing the wall with your feet about 45 cm (18 in) apart. **Standing facing your back with his feet between yours, he bends his knees and enters you from below.** Holding your hips to steady himself, he leans back while you lean forwards against wall, his hips pressed against your hips.

On the Move
Live life in the fast lane.
- **Do it on a roller coaster.** Studies show that screaming your head off on an amusement park ride causes a surge in adrenaline and endorphins, both of which give you a sexy thrill.
- **The seat belts in your car** can be used for light bondage at a pinch.

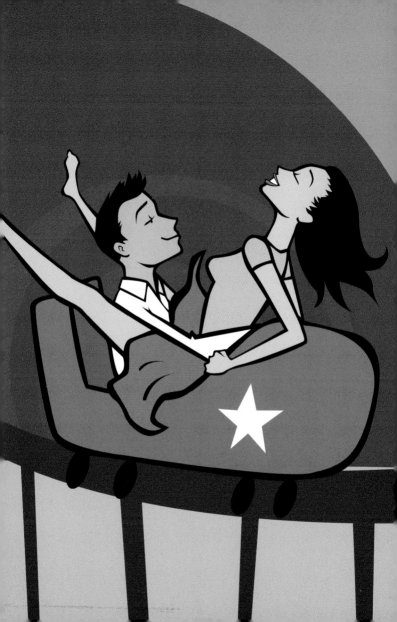

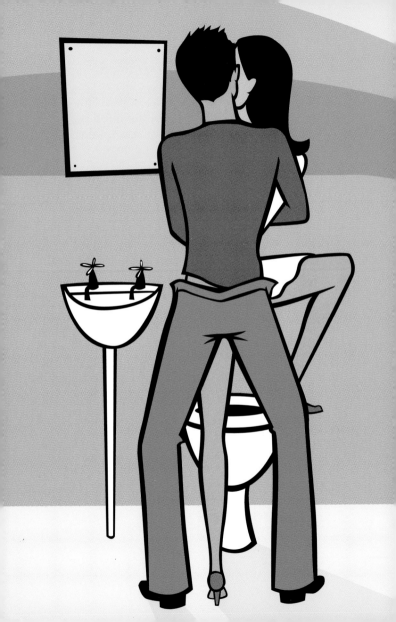

- If you indulge on the bonnet, **make sure the car alarm is off and the engine is cool.**
- Inside the car, **avoid unintentional pressing of the horn during the throes of abandonment** (drawing embarrassing attention to the vehicle) by jumping into the back seat. Another good car position is him sitting in the passenger seat with you on his lap facing him (if your legs are very long, you can rest them on his shoulders).
- While there's a lot to be said for a Porsche, according to the Petersen Auto Museum in Los Angeles, **the Volvo 70 Wagon is your best bet for quickie auto nookie** because of its frolic-friendly features: spacious, supple leather interior and rear seats that fold down to create a flat surface.
- **It's easy to hide a hand job under one of those little airplane blankets.** And if you're really sneaky, you can rest your head on your partner's lap and just happen to have oral sex. But try not to let your head bob up and down (unless there's turbulence).
- **Join the Mile High Club** (then you can register at www.milehighclub.com) by having sex on a plane once you reach cruising altitude. You can make a quick getaway to the toilet during the movie when there's usually no meal or beverage services. Face-to-face standing sex is best or he can enter you from behind (bonus: you can both watch in the mirror – see tip 96).

H2-Ohhh!

Make your own waves.

- **Hold on to your bikini bottoms.** You don't want to do the Walk of Shame back to your towel.
- The perfect pool or ocean water level is waist high (any lower and it's embarrassing, any higher and your passion may be swept away). **If you're surrounded by sunbathers, hold your breath and sink to the bottom,** pull your bikini bottoms to one side and let him perform oral thrill.
- **Have him stand up and enter you while you float on your back** – now try that when you're landlocked!
- In general, **the water needs to be quite warm so his erection won't sink.** However, the heat in a hot tub can cause blood vessels to dilate so his erection may not be as firm.
- While the beach seems movie-made for getting swept away, when sand gets in the creases and holds of the vagina, it can cause abrasions (think sandpaper), which makes it easier to catch STDs, including HIV.
- If possible, **have him enter you before you get wet and wild** so your natural wetness doesn't wash away first.

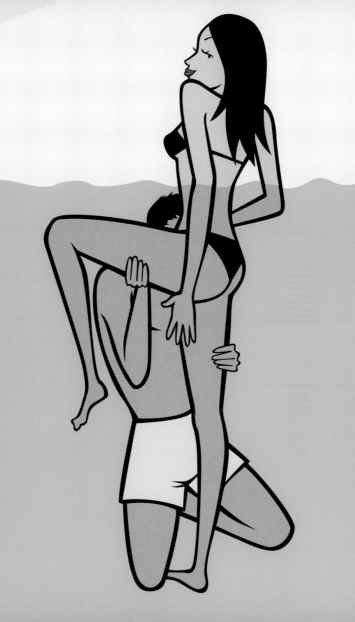

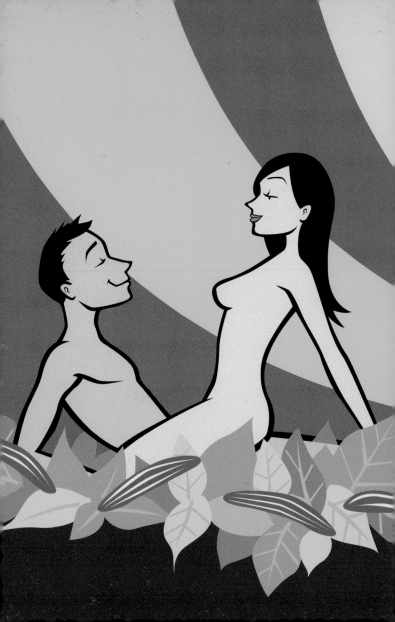

Going Green

Become a nature lover.

- Make use of the great outdoors. **Sunlight is additive-free Viagra.** One theory is that it makes people hornier because it suppresses their melatonin, a hormone believed to be the biological version of a five-course meal (in other words, it diminishes sexual desire). At the same time, it's speculated that sunshine increases serotonin and other hormones that make us more open to back-to-nature nookie.

- Do it in a cucumber patch – according to a study conducted by the Smell & Taste Treatment and Research Foundation, **the most arousing smell for women is cucumber** (lavender comes in second, great if you're in Provence).

- If passion overtakes you while you're walking in the woods, remember that mozzies love moist dark places – you get the picture (ouch!). **Spray yourselves with repellent before heading out.** A blanket or sleeping bag will also serve as barrier between you and any creepy crawlies.

- **Make sure you know what stinging nettles and poison ivy look like** (check out a website like www.vth.colostate.edu/poisonous_plants/).

- If you want extra wood, **choose a tree wider than your hips so it'll hold you up as you lean back against it.** If the bark is smooth, you can prop your bottom against it and wrap your legs around his waist so that it supports your weight.

85

On the Town
Make a break for it.

- **Hit the bathroom when you're at a restaurant.** The locked door won't arouse suspicion for at least 5 minutes (which is all you need). Also watching yourselves in the mirror as you go at it is pretty damned hot.
- **Go for the ladies' toilet,** as there is more privacy there than in the gents'.
- **If you do it in a dressing room, be careful about doing it against shoddy walls** (they may collapse). A changing bench or chair is much easier and won't arouse the suspicion of any curious salespeople.
- **You can have a quickie without leaving your table at a restaurant** if the tablecloth is long. Just use your big toe to masturbate each other.
- At the office, use a chair without wheels and flick on the computer monitor for sexy mood lighting (he sits and you perch on his lap).
- **If you're at a boring party, head for a tight closet.** He can squat on his knees while you lay on your back resting your knees on your chest and placing your feet on his torso. Start your motors. It's easy to get into and you get lots of deep thrusting.

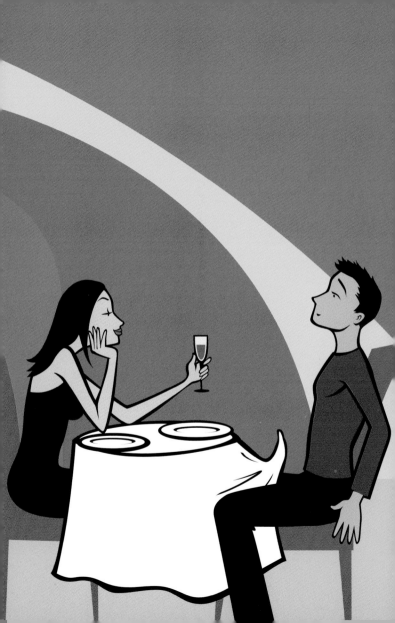

GET IN POSITION

The top moves to master for playing beat-the-clock sex.

Standing Up:

- It can be tricky to match up your love organs if you're different heights, so face away from him and **bend over so that your hands are flat on the floor and your weight is forwards** (or lean against a wall). He simply enters you from behind. Because all you have to do is slip down your knickers (or just wear crotchless), you can take this show on the road – your office desk, the restaurant toilet, wherever the urge strikes.
- Tip 91 (the position for the stairs) will also even things out.
- If he's strong and you're light, try what the *Kama Sutra* calls suspended congress: **while he leans back against a wall, you face him, sitting on his joined-together hands (he should lace his fingers), with your arms around his neck.** You can move yourself by extending your legs and putting your feet against the wall.

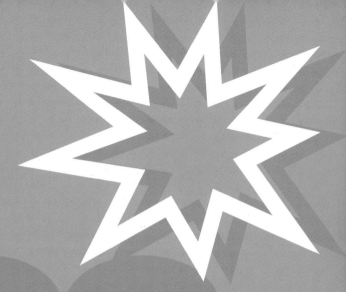

Some moves are two-in-one:

- **Anything rear entry gives the deep penetration often needed with quick sex** and lets his penis hit the ultrasensitive front of your vaginal wall.
- If you're sitting in a chair, face away from him, as he can then also massage your clitoris. **Hooking your leg over the chair leg will create extra friction between your clitoris and his penis.**

- **Keep your legs together:** This straight-laced position can trigger an instant orgasm by making it easier to clench your thigh muscles, which continue far up enough to stimulate your inner clitoris (the tissue actually extends 9 cm (3.5 in) – about the length of your middle finger – up into the pelvic area).
- **Wear a girdle – sexy – yes!** It puts pressure on the lower abs, which stimulates your inner clitoris (see above). Or get him to use his hand – anything that presses down on the part of your abs just above your pubic mound (his hand, your hand, a stack of bricks) during intercourse should do the trick because it sandwiches your inner clitoris between the proverbial rock and a hard place – in this case, your tensed muscles and his penis. **Extra tip – make sure he's inside you first as it will be difficult for him to hit the mark otherwise.**

The door jamb: Make use of the entryways to both your body and home with this position (part of the appeal is you may get busted by neighbours or flat-mates). Caution: don't wear socks, it can make things uncomfortably slippery. **Find a narrow doorway. He leans backwards against the door jamb while you do the same with the other, straddling him.** You can figure out the rest.

The One-Minute: So-called because that's all he'll be able to hold it for unless he's Arnie Schwarzenegger. He sits down with his legs bent and his feet flat on the floor and his hands on the ground behind him. He pushes his bottom up off the floor, supporting his weight with his arms and legs. You mount, crouching over him, and ride off into the sunset (good for you're doing tip 82).

HOME SWEET HOME

Listen to your mother's advice: Get out of bed!

- **Have sex sitting on or leaning against a washing machine** during the spin cycle for an extra orgasmic spin.
- **The nozzle at your kitchen sink** will add new meaning to the phrase, 'getting hosed' when used during a quickie.
- Handy for sex in the kitchen or any other confined space is **sitting face-to-face and wrapping your legs around his waist** and your arms around his neck.
- **If you stop on the stairs,** stand one step higher to make penetration a snap.
- **Straight-back chairs give more room for manoeuvring.** You can sit on his lap facing away from him or wrap your legs around him facing him. Or kneel on the chair holding onto the back (though you may topple over if things get vigorous – which we hope they will).

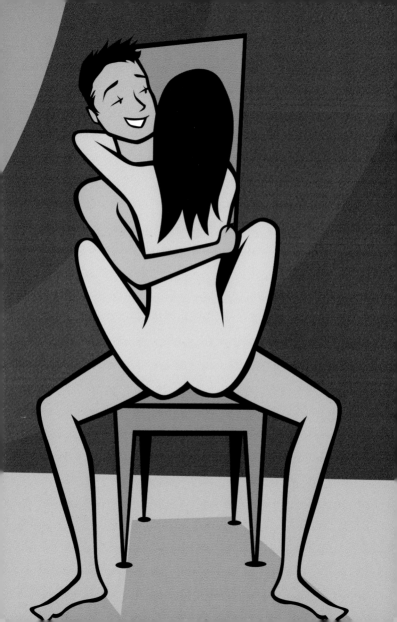

Minute Five:
Oh!

You might think that all it takes to have a quickie is a penis, a vagina and a few minutes. Not so fast.

Here is something you don't know: Erogenous zones – dense nerve endings – crackle all over the body, particularly in the earlobes, neck, palms, inner thighs and the backs of the knees. In one study, women were able to orgasm simply from having their arms stroked.

Men's and women's bodies have roughly the same landscape of nerve endings, meaning there's a whole continent of hot spots out there for the taking. The quickie is ideally suited for starting your pleasure expedition. Since you need to move quickly, here's your love map for increasing your thrill power in a hurry. Get ready to spin your orgasms into roargasms.

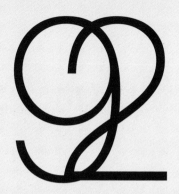

JUST DO IT

New 5-second tricks for packing 30 minutes of lovemaking into 5.

Talk dirty: Tell your lover what you want. Explicitly. Some suggestions: 'Mmm, squeeze my nipple. Harder. Yes, that feels so good' – and so on. You get the idea. This isn't just to turn him on (though that's definitely a blissful side effect). But according to a *Journal of Sex and Marital Therapy* study, **women who can talk freely about sex have a higher degree of sexual satisfaction than those who can't.** Now that should get you saying 'Yes, yes, yes!'

93 Go for his jugular: **There is evidence that the physiological state of sexual arousal is similar to the physiological stress state of fear, anxiety or threat.** In each of these states, blood pressure rises, the pulse quickens, adrenaline is released into the system and the body is energized and alert. Physically, the body is primed, and it may be possible to transform that primed state into a frenzy of sexual excitement.

94 Be selfish: Remember all that stuff your mother taught you about being polite? Forget it. This is no time to worry about the other guy. A quickie is every man and woman for himself and herself in a mad thrash for ecstasy. If you're thinking about pleasing him or he's thinking about satisfying you, then you're both missing the point. **Don't think about anything except giving yourself pleasure** (see tips 71 to 73 to get you on the me-me-oh-me road).

95

According to one poll, 40 per cent of men questioned are turned gooey by the natural scent of your nether regions. Not surprising since your vagina is a potent source of pheromones, chemicals that attract the opposite sex. Use it to your advantage – **touch your vagina and bring the scent to your partner's nose for a guaranteed turn-on.**

96

Use your eyes as well as your hands and mouth. A 1986 Archives of Sexual Behavior study reveals that both men and women are stimulated by erotic images, so keep the lights on and your eyes wide open.

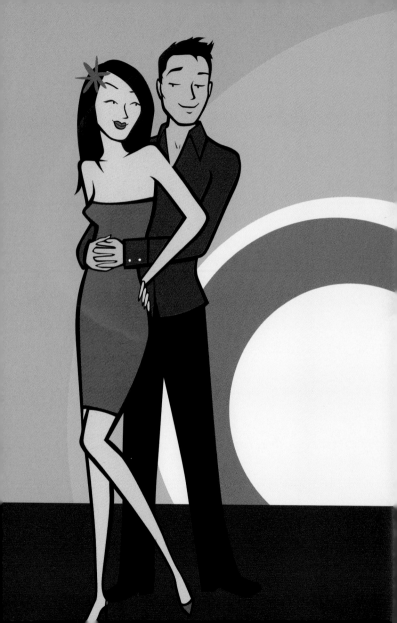

Pump up his passion by playing him a subliminally sensual tape of his favourite tunes (see tip 43 for which sounds to groove to). **Music actually activates the pleasure circuits of the brain** – the response can be so strong that it can even be orgasmic, according to a McGill University study on the subject.

97

8

Become a lady in red. **The colour crimson is reputed to amp up passion and enthusiasm,** so wear it when you want some feel-good fire.

LET YOUR FINGERS DO THE WALKING

To make the most of your time, here are a few pointers to keep at your (and his) fingertips.

Temples: Press your partner's temples and you'll feel veins throbbing. This pleasure point seems to have a direct link with the hypothalamus, your brain's bliss centre.

Ears: The cliché of blowing in your lover's ear is dead-on accurate. Stimulation from a darting tongue or a light, probing finger is such a powerful aphrodisiac that it can bring some men to orgasm. Researchers call the phenomenon the auriculogenital reflex and trace its origins to a nerve in the ear canal.

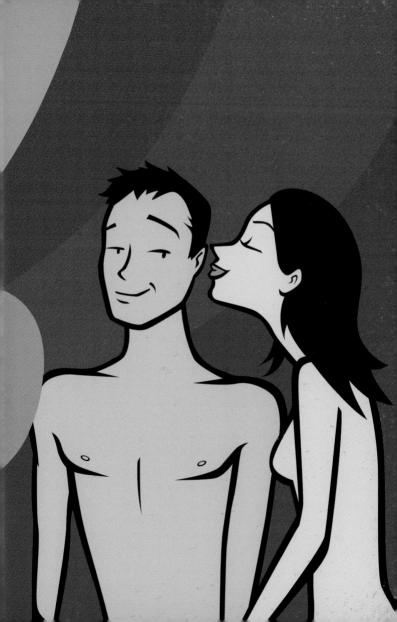

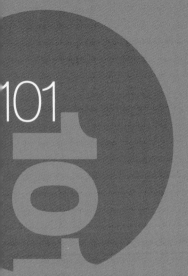

Mouth: When following tip 118, trace the outline of your partner's lips. He'll feel a familiar zing when you reach the corner of his mouth. This area is packed with rarely reached nerves just longing for some good loving.

Neck and spine: Try quick, playful love bites, especially on the ultra-sensitive collarbone. Move towards the centre of the back and trace the contours of the spine lightly with your tongue. Travel up and down your partner's back, blowing and tickling lightly as you go and watch him arch with pleasure.

Underarms: The tremendous accumulation of nerve endings here makes for great erotic potential. For a go-weak-at-the-knees move, use only your fingertips to stroke lightly and rhythmically from the rib cage towards the arms.

Nipples: You know that yours like attention, but so do his. Researchers have discovered that men's breasts have the same potential for erotic pleasure as women's breasts. In both sexes, the breasts are richly supplied with nerve endings, especially in the nipple area. Although only half as many men as women get hard nipples spontaneously when aroused, men's nipples are about as likely as women's to become erect when directly stimulated, and the sensation can sometimes make him explode.

Belly Button:
Anthropologists call
it a 'genital echo',
meaning its shape
reminds us of the
vaginal opening,
turning it into an
instant visual turn-on.
Heighten the carnal
pleasure by probing it
with a darting tongue
while tracing the outline
with your index finger.

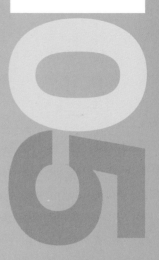

Lower Belly: There
is an erogenous
connection between
the belly button and
pubic patch, marked
out by a sensitive
south-of-the-navel
hairline. It will feel
fantastic when stroked.
Happy Trails.

107

Inner Thighs: This patch of land is ablaze with nerve endings because of the proximity to the genitals. Start with strokes so light that they barely register on your fingertips, and build to a crescendo of long, powerful strokes that work your fingers deep into the tender thigh muscles. Wowza.

108

Knees: The tender flesh behind the knee is good for both a tickle and a turn-on. Make sure your partner's leg is fully extended, then gently trace a figure-eight on the back of the knee with your fingertips or the tip of your tongue.

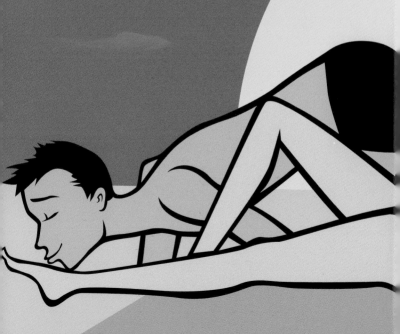

109

Fingers and Toes: Yes, it's true. Suck away. And don't forget to use your tongue to probe the crevices between each and every digit (on second thought, this might be best when doing tip 84 to keep things spic 'n span).

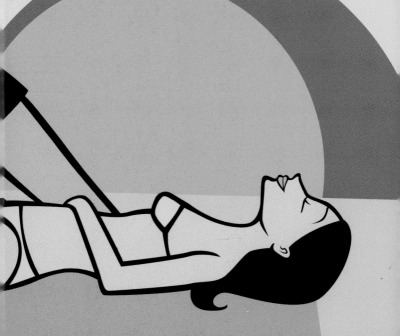

GOING DOWNTOWN

Measure for measure the muscle in your mouth holds more potential for pleasure than the one between your legs (and that goes for him, too).

Take a sip of water to **keep your mouth – and things – wet and shiny** (see tip 42).

Vary the temperature: Sip a hot drink or keep an ice cube in your mouth.

To speed things up, **let your mouth and hands work together.**

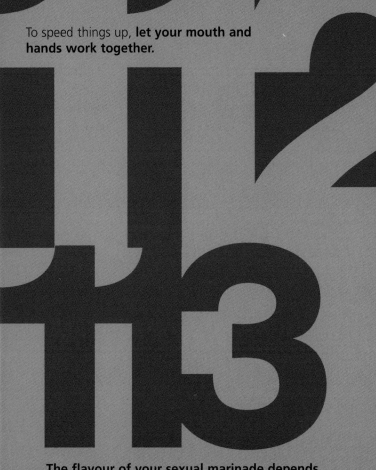

The flavour of your sexual marinade depends on your diet: Cow chompers have a pungent zest, vegetarians have a subtler flavour, spice lovers will pack a potent punch and the booze and ciggie brigade will have a slightly sour taste.

Hum.

Men tend to use their tongues like a mini penis. Instead, give him a new mental image with three words: ice scream cone.

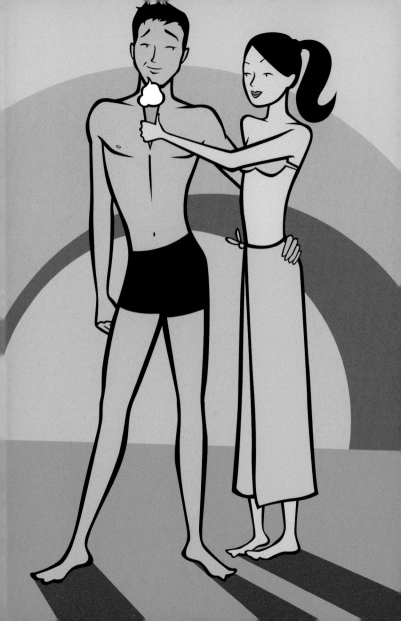

A DIRECT HIT

Ultimately, you will need to focus – these sex-marks-the-spots are guaranteed to get your erotic juices flowing.

4 ways to work his penis (he'll be your love slave forever):

- **Don't rush when giving him a hand-job.** Going at warp speed will sometimes kill the sensation for him, so take it down a notch (in the time it takes to say 'Mississippi', you should go up and down about two times).
- Most women use a simple up-and-down stroke with the thumb pointing up for a hand-job. **Instead, start with the thumb pointing down and stroke up.** When you get to the head, flip your hand over and go down. Then switch to the other hand.
- The V-Spot: There's a V-shaped break in the ridge that runs around the head of his penis – **this is a small patch of skin can bring mind-blowing bliss** (just think of him stroking your clitoris).
- **The blood vessel-like seam on the underside of his penis that runs from just below the shaft to halfway down the scrotum is his scream seam.** Massaging it will directly massage his urethra – a supersensitive tube that is capable of registering intense pleasure.

Here's how to make it happen every time:
- On him: **Poke his perineum (the thumbnail-sized dimple just behind his scrotum).**
- On you: **Clitoris, clitoris, clitoris** – like the estate agents say, it's all about location. But there are also points inside the vagina that get hot when pressed – the G-spot (one-third of the way up the canal on the front wall), the AFE zone (another third up – stimulation of this spot also helps lubrication and sometimes leads to multiple orgasms) and the cervix (the lump-like opening to the uterus at the end of the canal).

SPEED BUSTERS

You can go from 1,000 to less than zero on the thrillometre in less time than it takes to say, 'Ouch'. Since you may not have time to restart your play, here's what to avoid in the first place.

Not kissing first: Avoiding the lips and diving straight for the erogenous zones gives the experience a pay-by-the-hour feeling where you're trying to get your money's worth by cutting out nonessentials. Of course, this may be the effect you're going for.

Breaking contact: The biggest downer to having a quickie is the lack of intimacy. Always keeping in touch with your partner's body makes a big difference. Move your hands together, or stroke them one at a time, in a continual flow. If you have to stop, keep one hand gently resting against your partner's body.

120

Not taking the extra minute to get hot and sweaty (see tip 42).

121

Yes, there's tip 21. **But you can still go too hard.** If he bashes his hip bones into your thigh or stomach, the pain is equal to two weeks of strenuous exercise concentrated into a few seconds.

122

Positioning yourselves incorrectly. The missionary position limits your clitoral stimulation, as well as your ability to move around beneath his body. Review tips 88 to 91 for the most spine- (and other bits) tingling moves on the run.

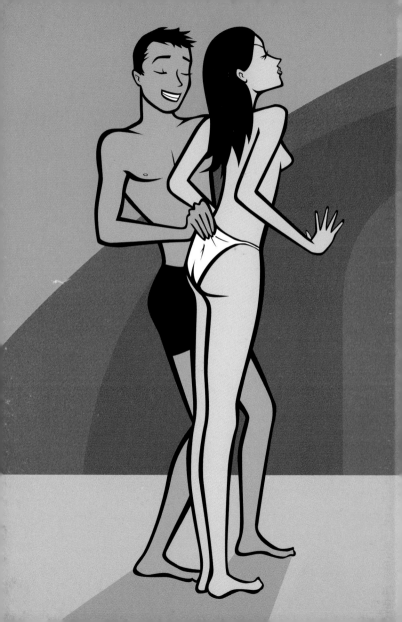

Giving a wedgie during foreplay. **Stroking gently through panties can be very sexy.** Pulling the material up between the thighs and yanking it back and forth in your rush to get on with the action is not.

123

124

Getting a non-battery powered vibrator (you don't want to waste precious minutes looking for a convenient outlet).

125

Forgetting, in your haste, to use any birth control.